The 1000 Workout Exercises Book

for Men and Women

The 1000 Workout Exercises Book for Men and Women

1000 Workouts to Build Muscle and Lose Fat

Extra Logging Sheets (electronic format) & Videos to Watch Exercises <u>Are Available by a Scanning QR Code</u>

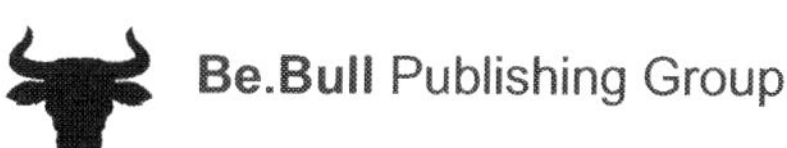

Be.Bull Publishing Group

Toronto, Canada

Authors:

Be.Bull Publishing Group
Devon Abbruzzese & Mauricio Vasquez

First Printing: March 2023

ISBN- 978-1-990709-66-1

FREE DOWNLOAD

BONUS No 1

Great news! You can access ALL the logging sheets from this book for FREE simply by scanning the QR code provided. Once you scan the code, you will have access to a Microsoft Excel sheet that you can easily download to your computer or laptop.

With this sheet, you have the flexibility to print additional copies of the workouts and continue recording your performance on those copies, or you can directly record your progress electronically on the sheet.

This way, you can keep track of your progress and monitor your growth. Don't miss out on this opportunity to take your fitness journey to the next level!

BONUS No 2

VIDEOS for ALL EXERCISES ARE AVAILABLE to check how the exercises are to be performed

(QR codes are found at the end of this book)

TIPS

- Adjust the weight of the kettlebell, the number of repetitions and the time cap for the workouts according to your capabilities, skills and physical condition
- Listen to your body and don't push yourself too hard
- If you don't have enough space where to run, you can do jumping jacks. 100-meter run is approximately equivalent to 50 jumping jacks
- Walk into the gym with a workout already selected for you
- Get motivated with a fun workout playlist
- Put your phone on airplane mode
- Start your workout with some stretches
- Pick the right weight - you will notice that the workouts don't indicate a specific weight. That is on purpose. Just choose a weight that is right for you.
- Log the details of each workout so you can track your progress. You can track the weight, time and number of repetitions
- Enjoy your workouts

Disclaimer

1. Be.Bull Publishing (Aria Capri International Inc.) strongly recommends that you consult with your physician before beginning any exercise program or workout. You should be in good physical condition and be able to participate in the exercises and workouts. We are not a licensed medical care provider and represents that we have no expertise in diagnosing, examining, or treating medical conditions of any kind, or in determining the effect of any specific exercise or workout on a medical condition.
2. You should understand that when participating in any exercise or workout, there is the possibility of physical injury. If you engage in the exercises and workouts of this book, you agree that you do so at your own risk, are voluntarily participating in these activities, assume all risk of injury to yourself, and agree to release and discharge Be.Bull Publishing (Aria Capri International Inc.) from any and all claims or causes of action, known or unknown, arising out of this book and videos.
3. The information provided through this book is not intended to be a substitute for professional medical advice, diagnosis or treatment. Never disregard professional medical advice, or delay in seeking it, because of something you have read on this book or watch in the videos. Never rely on information on this book or videos in place of seeking professional medical advice.
4. Be.Bull Publishing (Aria Capri International Inc.) is not responsible or liable for any advice, course of treatment, diagnosis or any other information, services or products that you obtain through this book or videos. You are encouraged to consult with your doctor with regard to the information contained on or through this book or videos. After reading this book or watching videos from this book, you are encouraged to review the information carefully with your professional healthcare provider.

If you purchased this book, I believe it's because you want to challenge yourself, be healthy and improve.

Keeping this in mind, I'm going to do a shameless plug here.

I think you might find this of value. Because body is important, but mind and spirit really matter too.

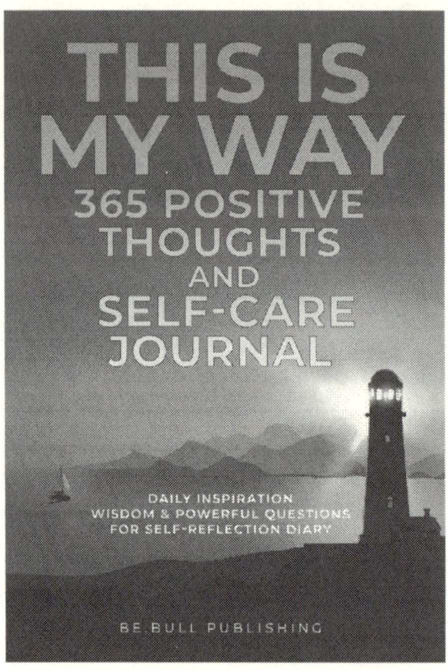

I recently published ***THIS IS MY WAY*** *journal.*

This is more than just a self-help book.

It is about a deeper understanding about life, who we are, and what our purpose is!

Discover the best version of ourselves and how to manifest that same improvement in all aspects of our life.

We are worth the 365-day investment and deserve the powerful results that will follow! This is one year of positive thinking for us.

To get a copy of this journal, scan this QR code.

Thank you,

Mauricio

If you want to add more variety to your workouts, scan this QR code to check these workout books!

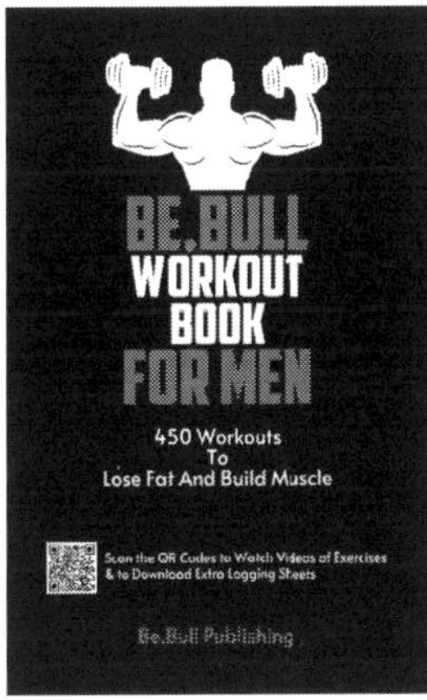

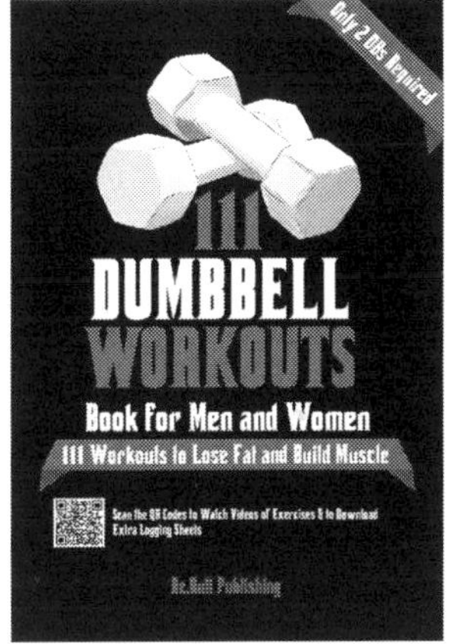

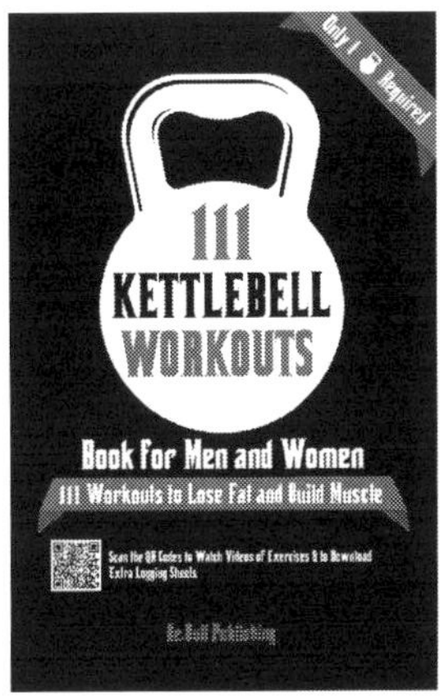

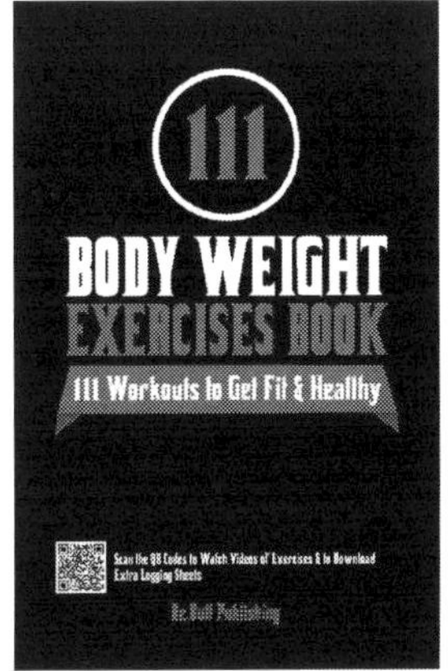

Dear valued customer,

We are a small family-owned business, and we'd like to please kindly ask you to leave us a review in Amazon by going to the link below or scanning the QR code

We don't have the same budget as big publishing companies, so your support would be really appreciated. Your feedback will mean a lot to us, and we thank you in advance!

Mauricio & Devon

		Day 1			Day 2			Day 3			Day 4			Day 5		
	WORKOUTS	Reps	Time	Weight	Reps	Time	Weight	Reps	Time	Weight	Reps	Time	Weight	Reps	Time	Weight
1	Complete as many rounds as possible in 12 minutes of:															
	- 3 Burpees															
	- 18 Push Presses															
	- 54 Single-unders															
2	Complete as many rounds as possible in 12 minutes of:															
	- 6 Squat Cleans															
	- 6 Pull-Ups															
3	For time:															
	- 2-minute Elbow Plank															
	- 10 Burpees															
	- 15 Kettlebell Swings															
	- 25 Push-Ups															
	- 35 Goblet Squats															
	- 35 Burpees															
	- 25 Kettlebell Swings															
	- 15 Push-Ups															
	- 10 Goblet Squats															
	- 2-minute Elbow Plank															
4	For time:															
	- 10 Turkish Get-Ups (Right Arm)															
	- 25 Kettlebell Swings															
	- 10 Overhead Squats (Left Arm)															
	- 25 Kettlebell Swings															
	- 10 Overhead Squats (Right Arm)															
	- 25 Kettlebell Swings															
	- 10 Turkish Get-Ups (Left Arm)															
5	12 Rounds for time of:															
	- 3 Air Squats															
	- 6 Dumbbell Push-Ups															
	- 12 Dumbbell Hang Squat Cleans															
6	3 Rounds for time of:															
	- 10 Dumbbell Man-Makers (Split reps between arms)															
	- 10 Burpees															
	- 500-meter Run															
	- 10 Air Squats															
	- 10 Hand-release Push-Ups															
7	3 Rounds for time of:															
	- 10 Bridge															
	- 10 Push-Ups															
	- 10 Air Squats															
	- 10 Bird Dog															
	- 10 Front Lunges															
	- 10 Downward dog to plank															
	- 10 Straight-Leg donkey kick															
8	10-9-8-7-6-5-4-3-2-1 Reps for time of:															
	- Hand-Release Push-Ups															
	- Air Squats															
	- Handstand Wall Walk															
9	For time:															
	- 100 Sit-ups															
	- 100 Spiderman Push-Ups															
	- 100 Air Squats															

		Day 1			Day 2			Day 3			Day 4			Day 5		
	WORKOUTS	Reps	Time	Weight	Reps	Time	Weight	Reps	Time	Weight	Reps	Time	Weight	Reps	Time	Weight
10	5 Rounds for time of:															
	- 20 Air Squats															
	- 20 Reverse Lunges (Alternating Legs)															
	- 20 Split Squat Jumps (Alternating Legs)															
	- 20 Squat Jumps															
11	As many rounds as possible in 10 minutes of:															
	- 10 Walkouts with Push-Ups															
	- 10 V-ups															
	- 10 Pistol Squats (Alternating Legs)															
12	Every minute on the minute for 21 minutes:															
	- Minute 1: 20 Push-Ups															
	- Minute 2: 20 V-ups															
	- Minute 3: 20 Air Squats															
	Repeat 7 times															
13	5 Rounds for time:															
	- 400-meter Run															
	- 20 Walking Lunges															
	- 5 Burpees															
14	4 Rounds for time of:															
	- 500-meter Run															
	- 20 Box Jumps															
15	As many reps as possible in 20 minutes:															
	- 5 Deadlifts															
	- 10 Box Jumps															
	- 15 Push-Ups															
16	For time:															
	- 30 Lunges (Alternating Legs)															
	- 15 Burpees															
	- 20 Kettlebell Swings															
	- 15 Burpees															
	- 10 meter Bear Crawl															
	- 15 Burpees															
	- 20 Kettlebell Swings															
	- 15 Burpees															
	- 30 Lunges (Alternating Legs)															
	- 15 Burpees															
	- 40 Sit-Ups															
	- 15 Burpees															
	- 50 Air Squats															
17	21-15-9 Reps for time:															
	- Burpees															
	- Kettlebell Swings															
18	For time:															
	- 100 Kettlebell Swings															
	- 100 Air Squats															
	- 100 Sit-Ups															
	- 100 Push-Ups															
19	For time:															
	- 100 Kettlebell Clean-and-Presses (Alternating arms)															
	- 3 Burpees at the top of each minute															
20	3 Rounds for time of:															
	- 15 Goblet Squats															
	- 30 Push-Ups															
	- 50 Sit-Ups															
	- 30 Russian Kettlebell Swings															
	- 15 Burpees															
	For time:															
	- 30 Burpees															

		Day 1			Day 2			Day 3			Day 4			Day 5		
	WORKOUTS	Reps	Time	Weight	Reps	Time	Weight	Reps	Time	Weight	Reps	Time	Weight	Reps	Time	Weight
21	- 60 Push-Ups															
	- 90 Kettlebell Swings															
	- Buy-in: 70 Sit-Ups															
22	For time:															
	- 1000-meter Run															
	- 50 Russian Kettlebell Swings															
	- 25 Air Squats															
23	10 Rounds for time of:															
	- 200-meter Run															
	- 15 Deadlift															
24	3 Rounds for time of:															
	- 500-meter Run															
	- 30 Dumbbell Squat Cleans															
25	10 Rounds for time of:															
	- 10 Dumbbell Man-Makers (Split reps between arms)															
	- 10 Dumbbell Deadlifts															
26	For time:															
	- 10 Burpees															
	- 30 Dumbbell Deadlifts															
	- 10 Burpees															
	- 30 Dumbbell Cleans															
	- 10 Burpees															
	- 30 Single-Arm Dumbbell Strict Presses (Split reps between arms)															
	- 10 Burpees															
	- 30 Dumbbell Thrusters															
	- 10 Burpees															
	- 30 Dumbbell Sumo Deadlift High-Pulls															
	- 10 Burpees															
	- 30 Dumbbell Snatches (Left Hand)															
	- 10 Burpees															
27	1-3-5-7-9-11-13-15 Reps for time of:															
	- Dumbbell Clusters (Dumbbell Clean + Dumbbell Thrusters)															
	- 100-meter Run															
28	For time:															
	- 100 Dumbbell Hang Clean Thrusters															
29	21-12-9 Reps for time of:															
	- Dumbbell Thrusters															
	- Burpees															
	- Air Squats															
30	5 Rounds for time of:															
	- 10 Dumbbell Power Snatches (Per arm)															
	- 10 Dumbbell Thrusters															
	- 10 Push-Ups															
31	40-20-10 Reps for time of:															
	- Air Squats															
	- Burpees															
	- Push-Ups															
	- Sit-Ups															
32	5 Rounds for time of:															
	- 10 Sit-ups															
	- 50 Jumping Jacks															
	- 10 Burpees															
	- 50 Jumping Jacks															
	- 10 Air Squats															
	- 50 Jumping Jacks															
	- 10 Hand Release Push-Ups															
	- 50 Jumping Jacks															
33	10 Rounds for time of:															
	- 10 Hand-Release Push-Ups															
	- 20 Walking Lunges (Alternating Legs)															
	- 30 Sit-Ups															

		Day 1			Day 2			Day 3			Day 4			Day 5		
	WORKOUTS	Reps	Time	Weight	Reps	Time	Weight	Reps	Time	Weight	Reps	Time	Weight	Reps	Time	Weight
34	As many rounds as possible in 20 minutes of: - 20 Front Lunges (Alternating Legs) - 25 Push-Ups - 30-second Up and down plank															
35	5 Rounds for time of: - 10 Push-Ups - 20 Sit-ups - 30 Air Squats															
36	For time: - 20 Burpees - 20 Jumping Jacks - 15 Burpees - 15 Jumping Jacks - 10 Burpees - 10 Jumping Jacks															
37	As many rounds as possible in 12 minutes of: - 5 Push Presses - 10 Deadlifts - 15 Box Jumps															
38	5 Rounds for time of: - 20 Air Squats - 15 Hand Release Push-Ups - 10 Burpees															
39	3 Rounds for time of: Round 1: - 30 Air Squats - 20 Jumping Jacks - 10 Push-Ups Round 2: - 30 Mountain Climbers - 20 Jumping Jacks - 10 Push-Ups Round 3: - 30 Bicycle Crunches - 20 Jumping Jacks - 10 Hand-Release Push-Ups															
40	As many reps as possible in 20 minutes: - 5 Dumbbell Man-Makers - 5 Box Step ups															
41	As many reps as possible in 15 minutes: - 60 Jumping Ropes - 15 Power Snatches															
42	Every minute on the minute for 15 minutes: - 5 Burpees - 5 Thrusters															
43	For time: - 100 Curtis p's - one "curtis p" complex is comprised of one power clean, one lunge (each Leg), and one push press.															
44	As many reps as possible in 15 minutes: - 5 Pendlay Rows - 10 Front Squats - 15 Push-Ups															
45	Complete as many rounds as possible in 20 minutes of: - 20 Bench Presses - 20 Pull-Ups - 20 Sit-ups															
46	For time of: 10,9,8...3,2,1 - Chest-to-Bar Pull-Ups															

		Day 1			Day 2			Day 3			Day 4			Day 5		
	WORKOUTS	Reps	Time	Weight	Reps	Time	Weight	Reps	Time	Weight	Reps	Time	Weight	Reps	Time	Weight
46	- Box Jumps - Straight Leg Sit-ups															
47	5 Rounds for time: - 15 Burpee - 15 Air Squat - 15 Hand Release Push-Ups															
48	As many reps as possible in 15 minutes: - 20 Box Jump - 15 Push Presses - 10 Pull-Ups															
49	For time: 21-15-9 - Kettlebell Swing - Push-Ups															
50	5 Rounds for time: - 10 Kettlebell Squats - 10 Burpees - 10 Kettlebell Swings - 10 Push-Ups															
51	As many rounds as possible in 15 minutes: - 25 Kettlebell Deadlifts - 25 Air Squats - 25 Tricep Dips															
52	Every minute on the minute for 10 minutes: - Even minutes - 20 Kettlebell Swings - Odd minutes - 10 Burpees															
53	For time: - 500-meter Run - 25 Push-Ups - 500-meter Run - 50 Goblet Squats - 500-meter Run - 25 Push-Ups															
54	As many rounds as possible in 20 minutes: - 5 Kettlebell Half Snatches (Right arm) - 5 Burpees - 5 Kettlebell Half Snatches (Left arm) - 5 Sit-ups															
55	As many rounds as possible in 15 minutes: - 10 Push-Ups - 20 Kettlebell Squats - 30 Mountain Climbers															
56	7 Rounds for time: - 7 Air Squats - 7 Kettlebell Deadlifts - 7 V-ups - 7 Push-Ups															
57	4 Rounds for time: - 20 Single-Arm Kettlebell Swings (Split reps between arms) - 20 Burpees - 20 Single-Arm Kettlebell Overhead Squats (Split reps between arms)															
58	As many rounds as possible in 15 minutes: - Kettlebell Power Snatches (Alternatig arms)															
59	21-19-17-15-13-11-9-7-5-3 Reps for time: - Burpees - Russian Kettlebell Swings															
60	10-9-8-7-6-5-4-3-2-1 Reps of: - Dumbbell Snatches (Per arm) - Hand-release Push-Ups															

	WORKOUTS	Day 1			Day 2			Day 3			Day 4			Day 5		
		Reps	Time	Weight	Reps	Time	Weight	Reps	Time	Weight	Reps	Time	Weight	Reps	Time	Weight
61	For time:															
	- Every minute on the minute for 3 minutes:															
	- 16 Dumbbell Rows (Split reps between arms)															
	- 10 Push-Ups															
	- Every minute on the minute for 3 minutes:															
	- 14 Dumbbell Rows (Split reps between arms)															
	- 10 Push-Ups															
	- Every minute on the minute for 3 minutes:															
	- 12 Dumbbell Rows															
	- 10 Push-Ups															
	*Then, As many rounds as possible in 3 minutes of:															
	Dumbbell Rows															
62	4 Rounds for time of:															
	- 400-meter Run															
	- 40 Dumbbell Deadlifts															
	- 40 Sit-Ups															
63	For time:															
	- 50 Dumbbell Power Snatches (Split reps between arms)															
	- 25-meter Dumbbell Overhead Walking Lunges (Per arm)															
	- 40 Dumbbell Overhead Squats (Alternate arms every 10 reps)															
	- 25-meter Dumbbell Overhead Walking Lunges (Per arm)															
	- 30 Dumbbell Hang Clean-and-Jerks (Alternate arms every 5 reps)															
	- 25-meter Dumbbell Overhead Walking Lunges (Per arm)															
	- 20 Dumbbell Squat Cleans															
	- 25-meter Dumbbell Overhead Walking Lunges (Per arm)															
	- 10 Dumbbell Squat Snatches (Split reps between arms)															
64	For time:															
	- 100 Double Dumbbell Ground-to-Overhead															
65	For time:															
	- 40 Dumbbell Thrusters															
	- 1000-meter Run															
	- 40 Burpees															
66	3 Rounds for time of:															
	- 30 Dumbbell Bicep Curls (Split reps between arms)															
	- 30 Dumbbell Strict Presses (Split reps between arms)															
	- 30 Dumbbell Lateral Raises (Split reps between arms)															
	- 30 Dumbbell Hammer Curls															
	- 30 Dumbbell UpRight Rows															
	- 30 Dumbbell Push Presses															
	- 30 Dumbbell Bicep Curls															
	2 Rounds for time of:															

	WORKOUTS	Day 1			Day 2			Day 3			Day 4			Day 5		
		Reps	Time	Weight	Reps	Time	Weight	Reps	Time	Weight	Reps	Time	Weight	Reps	Time	Weight
67	- 30 Dumbbell Squats - 30 Burpees - 300-meter Run - 30 Dumbbell Push Presses - 30 Lateral Jumps Over Dumbbells - 30 Dumbbell Power Cleans - 30 Dumbbell Lunges															
68	For time: - 30 Dumbbell Devil Presses - 60 Dumbbell Thrusters - 90 Burpees															
69	For time: - 11 Dumbbell Snatches (Left arm) - 11 Dumbbell Overhead Lunges (Left arm) - 11 Dumbbell Snatches (Right arm) - 11 Dumbbell Overhead Lunges (Right arm) - 11 Dumbbell Power Cleans (Left arm) - 11 Dumbbell Squats (Left arm) - 11 Dumbbell Power Cleans (Right arm) - 11 Dumbbell Squats (Right arm)															
70	5 Rounds for time of: - 20 Sit-ups - 60 Jumping Jacks - 20 Air Squats - 60 Jumping Jacks															
71	As many rounds as possible in 12 minutes of: - 20 Single-Leg Squats - 20 Push-Ups															
72	4 Rounds for time of: - 20 Reverse Lunges (Alternating Legs) - 40 Push-Ups - 60 Air Squats															
73	5 Rounds for time of: - 10 Handstand Push-Ups - 10 Sit-ups - 10 Air Squats - 10 Front Lunges (Alternating Legs)															
74	As many rounds as possible in 12 minutes: - 3 Burpees - 6 Push-Ups - 9 Mountain Climbers															
75	As many rounds as possible in 21 minutes: - 7 Air Squats - 14 Power Jacks - 21 Reverse Crunches															
76	For time: - 50 Air Squats - 25 Push-Ups - 50 Air Squats - 25 Push-Ups															
77	3 Rounds for time of: - 20 Air Squats - 20 Hand-Release Push-Ups - 20 Reverse Lunges (Alternating Legs) - 30-second Plan - 30 Jumping Jacks															
78	5 Rounds for time of: - 20 Air Squats - 20 Push-Ups															

		Day 1			Day 2			Day 3			Day 4			Day 5		
	WORKOUTS	Reps	Time	Weight	Reps	Time	Weight	Reps	Time	Weight	Reps	Time	Weight	Reps	Time	Weight
78	- 20 Front Lunges (Alternating Legs)															
	- 20 Mountain Climbers															
	- 20 Sit-ups															
79	For time:															
	- 100 Shoulder Taps															
	- 100 Sit-ups															
	- 100 Push-Ups															
	- 100 Air Squats															
80	15-13-11-9-7-5-3 Reps for time:															
	- Kettlebell Snatches (each arm, Alternating)															
	- After every round, perform:															
	- 5 Burpees															
	- 15 Prison Squats															
81	10 Rounds for time:															
	- 10 Kettlebell Squats															
	- 10 V-ups															
	- 10 Kettlebell Lunges															
82	For time:															
	- 400-meter Run															
	- 40 Russian Kettlebell Swings															
	- 40 Kettlebell Taters															
	- 300-meter Run															
	- 30 Russian Kettlebell Swings															
	- 30 Kettlebell Taters															
	- 200-meter Run															
	- 20 Russian Kettlebell Swings															
	- 20 Kettlebell Taters															
	- 100-meter Run															
	- 10 Russian Kettlebell Swings															
	- 10 Kettlebell Taters															
83	For time:															
	- 500-meter Run															
	- 20 Kettlebell Swings															
	- 20 Burpees															
	- 20 Air Squats															
	- 20 Single-Arm Kettlebell Push Press (Right arm)															
	- 500-meter Run															
	- 20 Kettlebell Swings															
	- 20 Burpees															
	- 20 Air Squats															
	- 20 Single-Arm Kettlebell Push Press (left arm)															
84	As many rounds as possible in 15 minutes of:															
	- 3 Burpees															
	- 6 Air Squats															
	- 9 Push-Ups															
	- 9 Kettlebell Squats															
85	As many rounds as possible in 15 minutes:															
	- 15 Kettlebell Deadlifts															
	- 50-meter Kettlebell Farmer's Carry (Right arm)															
	- 15 Kettlebell Thrusters															
	- 50-meter Kettlebell Farmer's Carry (Left arm)															
86	As many rounds as possible in 15 minutes:															
	- 5 Russian Kettlebell Swings															
	- 5 Burpees															

		Day 1			Day 2			Day 3			Day 4			Day 5		
	WORKOUTS	Reps	Time	Weight	Reps	Time	Weight	Reps	Time	Weight	Reps	Time	Weight	Reps	Time	Weight
	*Add 2 reps after each round															
87	For time:															
	- 5 Russian Kettlebell Swings															
	- 50-meter Kettlebell Farmer's Carry (Right arm)															
	- 50-meter Kettlebell Farmer's Carry (Left arm)															
	- 10 Alternating Single-Arm Kettlebell Swings															
	- 20 American Kettlebell Swings															
	- 50-meter Kettlebell Farmer's Carry (Right arm)															
	- 50-meter Kettlebell Farmer's Carry (Left arm)															
	- 10 Left-Arm Kettlebell Swings															
	- 10 Right-Arm Kettlebell Swings															
	- 50 Russian Kettlebell Swings															
88	For time:															
	- 25 Kettlebell Deadlifts															
	- 25 Push-Ups															
	- 25 Kettlebell Squats															
	- 25 Burpees															
	- 25 Kettlebell Swings															
89	6 Rounds for time:															
	- 12 Kettlebell Rows (Split reps between arms)															
	- 10 Push-Ups															
	- 12 Goblet Squats															
	- 12 Kettlebell Swings															
90	11 Rounds for time of:															
	- 1 Dumbbell Push-Up															
	- 1 Dumbbell Plank Row (Right-Arm)															
	- 1 Dumbbell Plank Row (Left-Arm)															
	- 1 Dumbbell Clean															
	- 1 Dumbbell Front Squat															
	- 1 Dumbbell Push Press															
	- 1 Dumbbell Overhead Reverse Lunge (Each Leg)															
91	For time:															
	- 500-meter Run															
	- 20 Dumbbell Clean and Presses															
	- 500-meter Run															
	- 20 Dumbbell Thrusters															
	- 500-meter Run															
	- 20 Dumbbell Burpees and Presses															
	- 500-meter Run															
92	For time:															
	- 1000-meter Run															
	- Max Dumbbell Thrusters															
	- 1000-meter Run															
93	For time:															
	- 1500-meter Run															
	*Then, 5 Rounds for time of:															
	- 20 Burpees															
	- 10 Dumbbell Snatches (Per arm)															
	- 10 Dumbbell Thrusters															
	- 21 Dumbbell Devil Presses															
	*Finally, perform:															
	- 500-meter Run															
94	10 Rounds for time of:															
	- 10 Dumbbell Lunges															
	- 10 Dumbbell Devil Presses															
	- 10 Air Squats															
	- 10 Push-Ups															
	- 10 Burpees															
	For time:															

		Day 1			Day 2			Day 3			Day 4			Day 5		
	WORKOUTS	Reps	Time	Weight	Reps	Time	Weight	Reps	Time	Weight	Reps	Time	Weight	Reps	Time	Weight
95	- 20 Burpees															
	- 1 Round of "Dumbbell DT"															
	- 15 Burpees															
	- 1 Round of "Dumbbell DT"															
	- 10 Burpees															
	- 1 Round of "Dumbbell DT"															
	- 5 Burpees															
	- 1 Round of "Dumbbell DT"															
	- 1 Round of "Dumbbell DT" consists of 12 Dumbbell Deadlifts, 9 Dumbbell Hand Power Cleans, and 6 Dumbbell Push Jerks															
96	For time:															
	- 10 Dumbbell Sit-Ups															
	- 10 Russian Twists with Dumbbell															
	- 10 Dumbbell Push Presses															
	- 10 Dumbbell Squats															
	- 10 V-Ups															
97	3 Rounds for time of:															
	- 10 Push-Ups															
	- 10 Dumbbell Hang Snatches (Split reps between arms)															
	- 10 Cossack Squats															
98	4 Rounds for time of:															
	- 10 Burpees															
	- 10 Dumbbell Hang Snatches (Split reps between arms)															
	- 10 Mantis Get-ups															
99	For time:															
	- 1000-meter Run															
	- 50 Dumbbell Devil Presses															
	- 1000-meter Run															
100	For time:															
	- 10 Dumbbell Power Snatches (Split reps between arms)															
	- 10 Dumbbell Renegade Rows (Split reps between arms)															
	- 10 Dumbbell Power Cleans															
101	3 Rounds for time of:															
	- 20 Dumbbell Lunges (Alternate Legs)															
	- 20 Dumbbell Snatches (Alternate arms)															
102	For time:															
	- 30 Burpees Over a Dumbbell															
103	3 Rounds for time of:															
	- 30 Dumbbell Hang Clean-and-Jerks (Alternate arms)															
	- 30 Dumbbell Squats															
104	3 Rounds for time of:															
	- 12 Dumbbell Sumo Squats															
	- 10 Arnold Press (Both arms)															
	- 10 Dumbbell Suitcase Lunges (Split reps between Legs)															
	- 10 Dumbbell Sit Up with Press															
	- 12 Half-Burpees Over Dumbbell															
105	For time:															
	- 500-meter Run															
	- 30 Dumbbell Squats															
	- 40 Burpees															
	- 50 Dumbbell Push Jerks															

		Day 1			Day 2			Day 3			Day 4			Day 5		
	WORKOUTS	Reps	Time	Weight	Reps	Time	Weight	Reps	Time	Weight	Reps	Time	Weight	Reps	Time	Weight
	- 15 Dumbbell Squats															
	- 20 Burpees															
	- 25 Dumbbell Push Jerks															
	<u>For time:</u>															
106	- 100 Jumping Jacks															
	- 200 Push-Ups															
	- 300 Air Squats															
	<u>For time:</u>															
	- 25 Jumping Jacks															
	- 250 Air Squats															
	- 25 Reverse Lunges (Alternating Legs)															
107	- 20 Hip extensions (Alternating Legs)															
	- 20 Forward Leg Swings (Alternating Legs)															
	- 20 Side Leg Swings (Alternating Legs)															
	- 20 Push-Ups															
	- 10 Jumping Lunges (Alternating Legs)															
	- 10 Spider-man steps															
	<u>Every minute on the minute for 16 minutes:</u>															
108	- 4 Burpees															
	- 4 Push-Ups															
	- 4 Tricep Dips															
	<u>For time:</u>															
	- 50 Air Squats															
109	- 50 Push-Ups															
	- 50 Air Squats															
	- 50 Push-Ups															
	<u>As many rounds as possible in 10 minutes of:</u>															
110	- 10 Air Squats															
	- 10 Push-Ups															
	- 10 Sit-ups															
	<u>5 Rounds for time:</u>															
	- Maximum Push ups															
111	- Maximum Sit-ups															
	- Maximum Air Squats															
	Rest 1 minute between rounds															
	<u>As many rounds as possible in 25 minutes:</u>															
	Round 1:															
	- 40 Plank jacks															
	- 30 Speed skaters															
	- 20 Russian Twists															
112	- 10 Reverse Crunches															
	Round 2:															
	- 40 Air Squats															
	- 30 High Knees															
	- 20 Jumping Jacks															
	- 10 Ups and down planks															
	<u>4 Rounds for time of:</u>															
	- 50 Jumping Jacks															
	- 20 Tricep Dips															
113	- 40 Squats															

		Day 1			Day 2			Day 3			Day 4			Day 5		
	WORKOUTS	Reps	Time	Weight	Reps	Time	Weight	Reps	Time	Weight	Reps	Time	Weight	Reps	Time	Weight
	- 50 Mountain Climbers															
	- 20 Modified v-Sits															
	- 20 Push-Ups with rotation															
	As many rounds as possible in 20 minutes of:															
	- 5 Sit-ups															
114	- 5 Hand Release Push-Ups															
	- 5 Reverse Crunches															
	- 5 Reverse Lunges (Per Leg)															
	3 Round for time of:															
	- 60 Jumping Jacks															
	- 30 Cross body punches															
115	- 30 Donkey Kicks (Alternating Legs)															
	- 30 Air Squats															
	- 30 Russian Twists															
	- 30 Bicycle Crunches															
	- 30 second Plank															
	With a Pair of Dumbbells, 4 rounds for time of:															
116	- 25-meter Weighted lunge															
	- 175-meter Farmers Carry															
	21-18-15-12-9-6-3 Reps for time:															
117	- Thrusters															
	- Bar Facing Burpees															
	As many reps as possible in 21 minutes:															
	from 0:00-07:00:															
	-1000-meter Run															
	- max Clean-and- Jerks															
	Rest from 07:00-10:00															
118	from 10:00-14:00:															
	- 800-meter Run															
	- max Power Snatches															
	Rest from 14:00-17:00															
	from 17:00-21:00:															
	- 400-meter Run															
	- max Thrusters															
	6 Rounds for time:															
119	- 9 Thruster															
	- 9 Pull-Ups															
	In 10 minutes, complete as much as possible of:															
	- 1 Deadlift															
	- 50-m Run															
	- 2 Deadlift															
120	- 100-m Run															
	- 3 Deadlifts															
	- 150-m Run															
	- 4 Deadlifts															
	- 200-m Run etc.															
	On a 25-minute clock, 5 rounds of:															
	- Row for 50 seconds, Rest 10 seconds															
	- Row for 40 seconds, Rest 20 seconds															
121	- Row for 30-second, Rest 30-second															
	- Row for 20 seconds, Rest 40 seconds															
	- Row for 10 seconds, Rest 50 seconds															
	For time:															
	- 40 Kettlebell Snatches															
	- 20-Calorie Ski															
	- 40 Kettlebell Goblet Squats															
122	- 20-Calorie Ski															
	- 40 Kettlebell Clean-and-Presses															
	- 20-Calorie Ski															
	- 40 Kettlebell Swings															

		Day 1			Day 2			Day 3			Day 4			Day 5		
	WORKOUTS	Reps	Time	Weight	Reps	Time	Weight	Reps	Time	Weight	Reps	Time	Weight	Reps	Time	Weight
	- 20-Calorie Ski															
123	For time:															
	- 30 Devil Presses															
	- 60 Dumbbell Thrusters															
	- 90 Burpees															
124	For time:															
	- 30 Walking Lunge Steps															
	- 30 Assisted Pull-Ups															
	- 30 Box Jumps															
	- 30 Single-unders															
	- 30 Back Extensions															
	- 30 Assisted Push-Ups															
	- 30 Hanging Knee Raises															
	- 30 Wall-Ball															
	- 30 Sit-ups															
	- 10 Rope Climbs															
125	For time:															
	- 35 Air Squats															
	- 35 Dumbbell Push Presses															
	- 35 Abmat Sit-up															
	- 35 Wall Ball Shots															
	- 35 Burpees															
	- 35 Med ball Twists															
	- 35 Push-Ups															
	- 35 Kettlebell Swings															
	- 35 Dumbbell Thrusters															
	- 400-meter Run															
126	20 Rounds for time:															
	- 18 Kettlebell Swings															
	- 6 Goblet Squats															
	- 3 Push-Ups															
127	50-40-30-20-10 Reps for time:															
	- Double-under															
	- Sit-ups															
128	10 Rounds for time:															
	- 30 Kettlebell Swings															
	- 30 Burpees															
	- 30 GHD Sit-ups															
129	Every minute on the minute in 21 minutes:															
	- minute 1: 20 Push-Ups															
	- minute 2: 25 Sit-ups															
	- minute 3: 35 Air Squats															
	repeat 7x															
130	For time:															
	- 400-meter Run															
	- 30 Wall-Ball Shots															
	- 200-Meter weighted Run															
	- 15 Wall-Ball shot															
	- 400-meter Run															
	- 400-meter Run															
	- 30 Wall-Ball Shots															
131	5 Rounds for time of:															
	- Max Planks															
	- 10 Squats															
	- 10 Front Lunges (Each Leg)															
	- 10 Push-Ups															
	- 10 Jumping Jacks															
	For time:															
	- 50 Jumping Jacks															
	- 5 Push-Ups															
	- 25 High Knees															
	- 10 Burpees															

	WORKOUTS	Day 1			Day 2			Day 3			Day 4			Day 5		
		Reps	Time	Weight	Reps	Time	Weight	Reps	Time	Weight	Reps	Time	Weight	Reps	Time	Weight
132	- 15 Crunches															
	- 10 Squats															
	- 5 Push-Ups															
	- 15 Crunches															
	- 5 Push-Ups															
	- 10 Squats															
	- 50 Jumping Jacks															
133	As many rounds as possible in 20 minutes of:															
	- 50 Jumping Jacks															
	- 40 Bicycle Crunches															
	- 30 Sumo Squats															
	- 20 Push ups															
	- 30 Jump Squats															
	- 40 Front Lunges (Alternating Legs)															
	- 50 Mountain Climbers															
134	4 Rounds for time of:															
	- 100 Jumping Jacks															
	- 10 Push-Ups															
	- 60-second High Knees (Alternating Legs)															
	- 30-second Mountain Climbers															
	- 30-second Plank															
135	As many rounds as possible in 12 minutes of:															
	- 3 Burpees															
	- 6 Push-Ups															
	- 9 Mountain Climbers															
	- 12 Tricep Dips															
136	As many rounds as possible in 12 minutes of:															
	- 3 Squats															
	- 6 Power Jacks															
	- 9 Push-Ups															
137	2 Rounds for time of:															
	- 60-second Up and down plank															
	- 50 Air Squats															
	- 40 Sit-ups															
	- 30 Glute bridges															
	- 20 Supermans															
	- 10 Squat Jumps															
	- 20 Supermans															
	- 30 Glute bridges															
	- 40 Sit-ups															
	- 50 Air Squats															
	- 60-second Plank															
138	5 Round for time of:															
	- 10 Half jacks															
	- 10 Plank jacks															
	- 10 Burpees															
	- 10 Push ups															
	- 10 Air Squats															
	As many rounds as possible in 25 minutes:															
	Round 1:															
	- 40 Mountain Climbers															
	- 30 Plan Shoulder Taps															
	- 20 Reverse Lunges															
	- 10 Push-Ups															
	Round 2:															

		Day 1			Day 2			Day 3			Day 4			Day 5		
	WORKOUTS	Reps	Time	Weight	Reps	Time	Weight	Reps	Time	Weight	Reps	Time	Weight	Reps	Time	Weight
139	- 40 Cross Jacks															
	- 30 Flutters Kicks															
	- 20 Squat to Front kick															
	- 10 Supermans															
	5 Rounds of:															
	- 10 Handstand Push-Ups															
	- 10 Jumping Jacks															
	- 10 Burpees															
	- 10 Tuck Jumps															
	- 10 Sit-ups															
140	For time of:															
	- 100 High Knees															
	- 90 Shoulder Taps															
	- 80 Air Squats															
	- 70 Butt Kicks															
	- 60 Leg Raises															
	- 50 Twist Crunches															
	- 40 Front Lunges (Alternating Legs)															
	- 30 Push-Ups															
	- 20 Russian Twists															
	- 10 Burpees															
141	As many rounds as possible in 15 minutes:															
	- 5 Air Squats															
	- 10 Hand Release Push-Ups															
	- 20 Bicycle Crunches															
	- 30 Cross Jacks															
142	2 Rounds for time of:															
	- 20 Push-Ups															
	- 30 V Sit-Ups															
	- 40 Jumping Jacks															
	- 50 Butt Kicks															
	- 60 Air Squats															
	- 50 Butt Kicks															
	- 40 Jumping Jacks															
	- 30 V Sit-Ups															
	- 20 Push-Ups															
143	As many rounds as possible in 10 minutes of:															
	- 30 Jumping Jacks															
	- 20 Air Squats															
	- 10 Push-Ups															
	- 30 Mountain Climbers															
	- 20 Front Lunges															
	- 10 Push-Ups															
144	For time:															
	- 100 Dumbbell Hang Clean Thrusters															
	- 5 Push-Ups to start, and at the end of each minute															
145	As many rounds as possible in 17 minutes of:															
	- 7 Dumbbell Goblet Thrusters															
	- 7 Dumbbell Power Snatches (Each arm)															
	- 7 Burpees															
146	As many rounds as possible in 16 minutes of:															
	- 6 Burpees															
	- 10 Hand-Release Push-Up															
	- 14 Dumbbell Goblet Squat															
	For time:															
	- 20 Air Squat Hops Over Dumbbell															

		Day 1			Day 2			Day 3			Day 4			Day 5		
	WORKOUTS	Reps	Time	Weight	Reps	Time	Weight	Reps	Time	Weight	Reps	Time	Weight	Reps	Time	Weight
	- 40 Dumbbell Shoulder to Overhead (Split reps between arms)															
	- 20 Air Squat Hops Over Dumbbell															
147	- 30 Dumbbell Squat Cleans (Split reps between arms)															
	- 20 Air Squat Hops Over Dumbbell															
	- 20 Dumbbell Thrusters															
	- 20 Air Squat Hops Over Dumbbell															
	- 10 Dumbbell Clusters															
	- 20 Air Squat Hops Over Dumbbell															
	<u>For time:</u>															
	- 30 Burpees															
148	- 30 Dumbbell Clean and Jerks															
	- 30 Dumbbell Snatches (Split reps between arms)															
	- 30 Burpees															
	<u>For time:</u>															
	- 30 Air Squat Hops Over Dumbbell															
	- 40 Dumbbell Shoulder to Overhead															
	- 30 Air Squat Hops Over Dumbbell															
	- 30 Dumbbell Squat Cleans															
149	- 30 Air Squat Hops Over Dumbbell															
	- 20 Dumbbell Thrusters															
	- 30 Air Squat Hops Over Dumbbell															
	- 10 Dumbbell Clusters (Dumbbell Clean + Dumbbell Thrusters)															
	- 30 Air Squat Hops Over Dumbbell															
	<u>For time:</u>															
150	- 10 Devil Presses															
	- 20 Dumbbell Lunges (Alternate Legs)															
	- 30 Dumbbell Push Presses															
	<u>5 Rounds for time of:</u>															
	- 10 Devil Presses															
151	- 20 Dumbbell Lunges (Alternate Legs)															
	- 10 Dumbbell Push Presses															
	- 20 Sit-Ups															
	<u>For time:</u>															
	- 1000-meter Run															
152	- 2 Rounds for time of:															
	- 12 Dumbbell Deadlifts															
	- 12 Dumbbell Swings															
	- 12 Dumbbell Thrusters															
	<u>12 Rounds for time of:</u>															
153	- 10 Dumbbell Hang Squat Cleans															
	- 10 Dumbbell Power Snatches (Split reps between arms)															
	<u>For time:</u>															
	- 20 Burpees															
	- 21 Dumbbell Snatches (Each arm)															
154	- 12 Dumbbell Thrusters															
	- 20 Burpees															
	- 21 Dumbbell Snatches (Each arm)															
	- 12 Dumbbell Thrusters															
	<u>For time:</u>															
	- 3 Dumbbell Hang Clean															
	- 4 Dumbbell Squats															
	- 5 Dumbbell Push Jerk															
	- 6 Bent Over Rows															
	- 7 Burpees															
	- 8 Dumbbell Thrusters															
155	- 9 Dumbbell Deadlifts															
	- 10 Dumbbell Snatches (Split reps between arms)															
	- 11 Dumbbell Swings															

	WORKOUTS	Day 1 Reps	Day 1 Time	Day 1 Weight	Day 2 Reps	Day 2 Time	Day 2 Weight	Day 3 Reps	Day 3 Time	Day 3 Weight	Day 4 Reps	Day 4 Time	Day 4 Weight	Day 5 Reps	Day 5 Time	Day 5 Weight
	- 12 Dumbbell Snatch To Reverse Lunge (Split reps between arms)															
	- 13 Dumbbell Devils Press															
	- 1000-meter Run															
156	For time:															
	- 15 Dumbbell Devil Presses															
	- 30 Air Squats															
	- 12 Dumbbell Devil Presses															
	- 30 Air Squats															
	- 9 Dumbbell Devil Presses															
	- 30 Air Squats															
	- 6 Dumbbell Devil Presses															
	- 30 Air Squats															
	- 3 Dumbbell Devil Presses															
157	For time:															
	- 50 Air Squats															
	- 50 Dumbbell Snatches (Alternate arms)															
	- 40 Air Squats															
	- 40 Dumbbell Snatches (Alternate arms)															
	- 30 Air Squats															
	- 30 Dumbbell Snatches (Alternate arms)															
	- 20 Air Squats															
	- 20 Dumbbell Snatches (Alternate arms)															
	- 10 Air Squats															
158	For time:															
	- 2 minute Max Dumbbell Renegade Rows															
	- 2 minute Max Push-Ups															
	- 2 minute Max Mountain Climbers															
	- 2 minute Max Air Squats															
	- 2 minute Max Dumbbell Power Snatches (Alternate arms)															
159	5 Rounds for time of:															
	- 10 Single-Arm Dumbbell Floor Press (Split reps between arms)															
	- 14 Russian Twists with Dumbbell															
	- 18 Dumbbell Windmill (Split reps between arms)															
	- 22 Dumbbell Sit-Up															
160	For time:															
	- 4 Dumbbell Renegade Rows															
	- 16 Dumbbell Snatches (Alternate arms)															
	- 24 Lateral Hops Over Dumbbell															
	- 4 Dumbbell Renegade Rows															
	- 16 Dumbbell Snatches (Alternate arms)															
	- 24 Lateral Hops Over Dumbbell															
161	For time:															
	- 500-meter Run															
	- 50 Kettlebell Single-Arm Hang Snatches (Split reps between arms)															
	- 500-meter Run															
	- 50 Kettlebell Single-Arm Hang Clean and Push Presses (Split reps between arms)															
162	As many rounds as possible in 15 minutes:															
	- 9 Sumo Deadlift High Pull															
	- 15 Goblet Squats															
	- 21 Kettlebell Swings															
	For time:															

		Day 1			Day 2			Day 3			Day 4			Day 5		
	WORKOUTS	Reps	Time	Weight	Reps	Time	Weight	Reps	Time	Weight	Reps	Time	Weight	Reps	Time	Weight
163	- 20 Turkish Get-Ups (Right Arm)															
	- 60 Kettlebell Swings															
	- 20 Overhead Squats (Left Arm)															
	- 60 Kettlebell Swings															
	- 20 Overhead Squats (Right Arm)															
	- 60 Kettlebell Swings															
	- 20 Turkish Get-Ups (Left Arm)															
164	For time:															
	- Every minute on the minute, perform Burpee(s). Start with 1 Burpee after minute 1, then 2 Burpees after minute 2, then 3 Burpees, etc.															
	(Stop adding Burpees once you get less than 30-second left for your Swings)															
165	As many rounds as possible in 15 minutes:															
	- 5 Burpees															
	- 10 Single-Arm Kettlebell Snatches (Each arm)															
	- 20 Lunges (Alternating Legs)															
166	4 Rounds for time:															
	- 400-meter Run															
	- 21 Kettlebell Swings															
	- 15 Burpees															
167	20- 18- 16-14-12-10-8-6-4-2 Reps for time of:															
	- Kettlebell Thrusters (Split reps between arms)															
	- Burpees															
168	50- 40-30-20-10 Reps for time of:															
	- Push-Ups															
	- Kettlebell Swings															
169	As many rounds as possible in 20 minutes:															
	- 500-meter Run															
	- 20 American Kettlebell Swings															
	- 15 Push-Ups															
	- 10 Burpees															
170	20- 18- 16-14-12-10-8 Reps for time:															
	- Kettlebell Thrusters (Split reps between arms)															
	- Kettlebell Deadlifts															
171	11-10-9-8-7-6-5-4-3-2-1-2-3-4-5-6-7-8-9-10 Reps for time:															
	- American Kettlebell Swings															
	- Burpees															
172	15-13-11-9-7-5-3-1 Reps for time:															
	-Kettlebell Taters															
	-Burpees															
173	20 Rounds for time:															
	- 15 Kettlebell Swings															
	- 10 Burpees															
174	For time:															
	- 400 Kettlebell Swings															

		Day 1			Day 2			Day 3			Day 4			Day 5		
	WORKOUTS	Reps	Time	Weight	Reps	Time	Weight	Reps	Time	Weight	Reps	Time	Weight	Reps	Time	Weight
	- 5 Burpees - every minute on the minute															
175	<u>5 Rounds for time:</u> - 6 Deadlifts - 6 Burpees - 5 Cleans - 5 Pull-Ups - 4 Thrusters - 4 Push-Ups															
176	<u>For time:</u> -50-40-30-20-10 -Kettlebell Swings -Kettlebell Goblet Squats															
177	<u>For Time:</u> - 12 Overhead Squats - 12 Chest-to-Bar Pull-Ups - 12 Jerks															
178	<u>As many rounds as possible in 15 minutes:</u> - 6 Russian Kettlebell Swings - 3 Burpees - 6 Cossack Squats (Alternating Legs) - 12 Russian Kettlebell Swings - 6 Burpees - 6 Cossack Squats (Alternating Legs)															
179	<u>10 Rounds for time:</u> - 10 Russian Kettlebell Swings - 5 Burpees - 10 American Kettlebell Swings - 5 Burpees															
180	<u>10 Rounds for time:</u> - 15 Russian Kettlebell Swings - 15 Push-Ups - 5 Burpees															
181	<u>21-15-9-9-15-21 Reps for time:</u> - Deadlifts - Burpees															
182	<u>As many reps as possible in 20 minutes:</u> - 10 Push Presses - 10 Kettlebell Swings - 15 Box Jumps															
183	<u>For time:</u> - 1000-meter Run - 30 Push-up then, 20 rounds of: - 3 Deadlift - 3 Clean-and-Jerks - 3 Front Squats then, perform: - 30 Push-Ups - 1000-meter Run															
184	<u>4 Rounds for time:</u> - 500-meter Run - 50 Push-Ups - 50 Sit-ups															

		Day 1			Day 2			Day 3			Day 4			Day 5		
	WORKOUTS	Reps	Time	Weight	Reps	Time	Weight	Reps	Time	Weight	Reps	Time	Weight	Reps	Time	Weight
	- 50 Air Squats															
	<u>For time:</u>															
	- 1000-meter Run															
185	- 21 Clean-and-Jerks															
	- 800-meter Run															
	- 21 Clean-and-Jerks															
	- 1000-meter Run															
	<u>For max reps of each:</u>															
	- 5 min. of Jumping Ropes															
	- 5 min. of Clean and Jerks															
186	- 3 min. of Jumping Ropes															
	- 3 min. of Clean and Jerks															
	- 1 min. of Jumping Ropes															
	- 1 min. of Clean and Jerks															
	<u>Buy in: 15 Devil Presses then, 3 rounds of:</u>															
187	- 12 Dumbbell Snatches															
	- 16 Toes to Bar - And cash out: 15 Devil Presses															
	<u>9 Rounds for time:</u>															
	- 9 Hang Power Cleans															
	- 9 Front Squats															
	- 9 Push Presses															
188	- 9 Burpees															
	- 9 Pull-Ups															
	- 9 Dips															
	- 9 Box Jumps															
	- 9 Sit-ups															
	<u>5 Rounds for time of:</u>															
	- Row 500 -meter															
189	- 10 Box Jumps															
	- 10 Deadlifts															
	- 10 Wall-Ball Shots															
	<u>For time:</u>															
	- 150 Double-unders															
	- 15-meter Single-arm Overhead Walking Lunges															
	- 25 Alternating Single-arm Dumbbell Thrusters															
190	- 15-meter Single- arm Overhead Walking Lunges															
	- 25 Alternating Single-arm Dumbbell Thrusters															
	- 15-meter Single- arm Overhead Walking Lunges															
	- 150 Double-unders															
	Time cap: 15 min															
	Run 2500 meters															
	<u>5 Rounds for time:</u>															
	- 1000-meter Row															
191	- 200-meter Farmer Carry															
	- 50-meter Waiter Walk, Right arm															
	- 50-meter Waiter Walk, Left arm															
	<u>For time:</u>															
192	- 2000 meter Row then, complete as many reps as possible of in 20 min:															
	- 5 Toes-to-Bars															
	- 10 Wall Ball Shots															
	- 15 Push-Ups															
	<u>As many reps as possible in 25 minutes</u>															

		Day 1			Day 2			Day 3			Day 4			Day 5		
	WORKOUTS	Reps	Time	Weight	Reps	Time	Weight	Reps	Time	Weight	Reps	Time	Weight	Reps	Time	Weight
193	- 5 Deadlifts															
	- 5 Hang Power Cleans															
	- 5 Front Squats															
	- 5 Push press															
	- 5 Back Squat															
194	For time:															
	- 20 Push-Ups, 1 Sit-up															
	- 19 Push-Ups, 2 Sit-ups															
	- 18 Push-Ups, 3 Sit-ups ...continue this pattern until...															
	- 2 Push-Ups, 19 Sit-ups															
	- 1 Push-Up, 20 Sit-ups															
195	For time:															
	- 1000-meter Run															
	- 100-Calorie Air Bike															
	- 100-Calorie Ski															
	- 100-Calorie Row															
	- 1000-meter Run															
196	As many reps as possible in 15 minutes:															
	- 10 Power Cleans															
	- 10 Burpees Over the Bar															
	- 20 Deadlifts															
	- 20 Pull-Ups															
197	Four 3-minute rounds of:															
	- Jog 100 meters with a medicine ball															
	- Max reps Wall-Ball Shots Rest 1 min. between rounds															
198	For time:															
	10 31 10 31 repo of:															
	- Wall Ball Shots															
	- Toes-to-Bars															
	- Burpees															
199	As many reps as possible in 10 minutes of:															
	- 15 Toes-to-Bars															
	- 10 Deadlifts															
	- 5 Snatches															
200	As many reps as possible in 12 minutes:															
	- 1-minute of Pull-ups															
	- 1-minute of Pull-ups															
	- 3-minute of Rowing															
	- 1-minute of Pull-ups															
	- 2 minute of Rowing															
	- 1-minute of Pull-ups															
	- 3-minute of Rowing															
201	As many reps as possible in 21 minutes:															
	- 11 Deadlifts															
	- 11 Wall Ball Shots															
	- 11 Toes-to-Bars															
	- 11 Hand Release Push-Ups															
202	5 Rounds for max reps:															
	- Hang Power Snatches															
	- Handstand Push-Ups															
	Rest as needed between rounds.															
203	6 rounds for time:															
	- 18 Calorie Assault AirBike															
	- 15 Air Squats															
	- 12 Sit-ups															
	For time:															

		Day 1			Day 2			Day 3			Day 4			Day 5		
	WORKOUTS	Reps	Time	Weight	Reps	Time	Weight	Reps	Time	Weight	Reps	Time	Weight	Reps	Time	Weight
204	- 30 High Knees															
	- 40 Squats															
	- 50 Jumping Jacks															
	- 60 Reverse Lunges (Alternating Legs)															
	- 70 Burpees															
	- 80 V-ups															
	- 90 Russian Twists															
205	For time:															
	- 20 Squats															
	- 20 Sit-ups															
	- 20 Push-Ups															
	- 20 Front Lunges (Alternating Legs)															
	- 20 Sit-ups															
	- 20 Reverse Lunges (Alternating Legs)															
	- 20 Push ups															
	- 20 Sit-ups															
	- 20 Push ups															
206	10 Rounds for time of:															
	- 10 Air Squats															
	- 10 Front Lunges (Alternating Legs)															
	- 10 Side Leg Swings (Each Leg)															
	- 10 Reverse Lunges (Alternating Legs)															
	- 10 Push-Ups															
207	5 Rounds for time of:															
	- 20 Crunches															
	- 25 Push-Ups															
	- 30 Jumping Jacks															
	- 35 Air Squats															
	- 45-second plank															
208	As many rounds as possible in 15 minutes of:															
	- 10 Power Jacks															
	- 10 Mountain Climbers															
	- 10 Curtsy Lunges															
	- 10 Speed skaters															
209	As many rounds as possible in 26 minutes of:															
	- 6 Dumbbell Devil Presses															
	- 6 Burpees Over Dumbbells															
	- 6 Dumbbell Thrusters															
210	As many reps as possible in 10 minutes of:															
	- 10 Dumbbell Thrusters															
	- 10 Burpee															
211	For time:															
	- 100 Dumbbell Thrusters															
	- 1 Burpee															
	- Keep adding 1 Burpee after every minute															
	For time:															
	- 30 Dumbbell Farmer's Carry (Alternate Lunges)															
	- 30 Push-Ups															
	- 30 Dumbbell Bent Over Rows															

		Day 1			Day 2			Day 3			Day 4			Day 5		
	WORKOUTS	Reps	Time	Weight	Reps	Time	Weight	Reps	Time	Weight	Reps	Time	Weight	Reps	Time	Weight
212	- 20 Dumbbell Farmer's Carry (Alternate Lunges)															
	- 20 Push-Ups															
	- 20 Dumbbell Bent Over Rows															
	- 10 Dumbbell Farmer's Carry (Alternate Lunges)															
	- 10 Push-Ups															
	- 10 Dumbbell Bent Over Rows															
	As many reps as possible in 10 minutes of:															
213	- 10 Dumbbell Deadlifts															
	- 10 Renegade Row (Alternate arms) with Pushup															
	5 Rounds for time of:															
214	- 30 Dumbbell Hang Squat Cleans															
	- 20 Burpees Over Dumbbell															
	As many rounds as possible in 25 minutes:															
	-First, 50-40-30-20-10 Reps for time of:															
	-Push-Ups															
215	-Kettlebell Swings															
	-Then, in the remaining time, as many rounds as possible of:															
	-Air Squats															
	As many rounds as possible in 15 minutes:															
	- 20 Kettlebell Swings															
216	- 15 Kettlebell Sumo Deadlift High Pulls															
	- 10 Kettlebell Goblet Squat															
	-Perform 5 Hollow Rocks every time you drop the Kettlebell															
	For time:															
	- 100-80-60- 40-20 Kettlebell Swings															
217	- 50-40-30-20-10 Air Squats															
	- 25-20-15-10-5 Burpees															
	- Alternating between Kettlebell Swings, Air Squats and Burpees															
	Every minute on the minute for 12 minutes:															
218	- Odd minute: 10 Kettlebell Thrusters (Split reps between arms)															
	- Even minute: 20 American Kettlebell Swings															
	5 Rounds for time:															
	- 22 Kettlebell Swings															
219	- 16 Kettlebell Power Cleans															
	- 10 Burpees															

	WORKOUTS	Day 1			Day 2			Day 3			Day 4			Day 5		
		Reps	Time	Weight	Reps	Time	Weight	Reps	Time	Weight	Reps	Time	Weight	Reps	Time	Weight
220	For time:															
	- 10 Kettlebell Snatches (Right-Arm)															
	- 10 Burpees															
	- 10 Kettlebell Snatches (Left-Arm)															
	- 30 Air Squats															
	- 15 Kettlebell Push Jerks (Right-Arm)															
	- 15 Burpees															
	- 15 Kettlebell Push Jerks (Left-Arm)															
	- 45 Air Squats															
	- 20 Kettlebell Cleans (Right-Arm)															
	- 20 Burpees															
	- 20 Kettlebell Cleans (Left-Arm)															
221	For time:															
	- 100 Air Squats															
	- 80 Kettlebell Swings															
	- 20 Push-Ups															
	- 20 Air Squats															
	- 60 Kettlebell Swings															
	- 20 Push-Ups															
	- 40 Air Squats															
	- 40 Kettlebell Swings															
	- 20 Push-Ups															
	- 60 Air Squats															
	- 20 Kettlebell Swings															
	- 20 Push-Ups															
	- 80 Air Squats															
222	For time:															
	- 60 Russian Kettlebell Swings															
	- 60 Russian Kettlebell Swings															
	- 50 Air Squats															
	- 40 Hand-release Push ups															
	- 50 American Kettlebell Swings															
	- 40 Lunges															
	- 30 Hand-release Push ups															
	- 40 Russian Kettlebell Swings															
	- 30 Air Squats															
	- 20 Hand-release Push ups															
	- 30 Kettlebell Swing Snatch (Split reps between arms)															
	- 20 Plyo Lunges															
	- 10 Hand-release Push ups															
223	For time:															
	- 120 Air Squats															
	- 80 Kettlebell Swings															
	- 20 Push-Ups															
	- 60 Air Squats															
	- 20 Push-Ups															
	- 40 Kettlebell Swings															
	- 20 Push-Ups															
	- 30 Air Squats															
	- 20 Kettlebell Swings															
	- 20 Push-Ups															
	- 15 Air Squats															
	- 10 Kettlebell Swings															
	- 20 Push-Ups															
	For time:															

		Day 1			Day 2			Day 3			Day 4			Day 5		
	WORKOUTS	Reps	Time	Weight	Reps	Time	Weight	Reps	Time	Weight	Reps	Time	Weight	Reps	Time	Weight
224	- Buy-In: 25 Burpees															
	- Then 10 Rounds of:															
	- 20 Kettlebell Swings															
	- 20 Push-Ups															
225	For time:															
	- 50 Russian Kettlebell Swings															
	- 50 Kettlebell Ballistic Rows (Split reps between arms)															
	- 20 Goblet Squats															
	- 50 Russian Kettlebell Swings															
	- 50 Kettlebell Push Presses (Split reps between arms)															
	- 50 Russian Kettlebell Swings															
	- 20 Goblet Squats															
226	For time:															
	- 2000 meter Run															
	- 50 Pull-Ups															
	- 50 Thrusters															
	- 2000 meter Row															
227	As many rounds as possible in 15 minutes of:															
	- 10 Hanging Knee Raises															
	- 20-Calorie Row															
	- 30 Push-Ups															
	- 20 Box Jumps															
	- 10 Pull-Ups															
228	6 Rounds for time:															
	- 21-Calorie Row															
	- 15 Burpee Box Jump Overs															
	- 9 Deadlifts															
229	For time:															
	- 2000 meter Row															
	- 1000-meter Run															
	- 2000 meter Row time cap: 25 minutes															
230	For time:															
	- 150 Squats															
	- 50 V-ups															
	- 120 Squats															
	- 40 V-ups															
	- 90 Squats															
	- 30 V-ups															
231	As many reps as possible in 21 minutes:															
	- 400-meter Run															
	- 21 Push-Ups															
	- 21 Box Jumps															
	- 15 Burpees															
	- 9 Pull-Ups															
232	2 Rounds for time:															
	- 10 Devil Presses															
	- 400-meter Run															
	- 30 Dumbbell sumo Cleans															
	- 300-meter Run															
	- 30 Dumbbell floor Presses															
	- 200-meter Run															

		Day 1			Day 2			Day 3			Day 4			Day 5		
	WORKOUTS	Reps	Time	Weight	Reps	Time	Weight	Reps	Time	Weight	Reps	Time	Weight	Reps	Time	Weight
	- 30 Dumbbell Front Squats															
233	5 Rounds for time: - 10 Deadlifts - 15-meter Single-arm Dumbbell Overhead Walking Lunges															
234	4 Rounds for time of: - Run 200-meters - 20 Kettlebell Swings - 10 Jumping Pull-Ups															
235	3 rounds for time of: - 50-ft. Overhead Walking lunge - 25 Sit-ups															
236	3 Round for time: - 30 Squat Cleans - 30 Pull-Ups - 800-meter Run															
237	For time: - 1000-meter Run - 10 Kettlebell Swings - 15 Burpees - 20 Wall Ball Shots - 25 Plate Overhead Lunges - 20 Toes-to-Bars - 15 Kettlebell Snatches - 10 Pull-Ups -1000-meter Run repeat back up the ladder to the top															
238	For time: - 50-meter Broad Jump - 25 Alternating Jumping Lunges - 250-meter Run															
239	As many reps as possible in 20 minutes: - 20 Sit-ups - 20 Devil Presses - 20 Alternating Dumbbell Lunges - 20 Dumbbell Push Presses															
240	For time: - 10 mile Run - 150 Burpee Pull-Ups															
241	5 Rounds for time: - 35 Double-unders - 5 Clusters - 1 Rope climb *1 Cluster is 1 clean and 1 Thruster															
242	As many reps as possible in 10 minutes: - 5 Deadlifts - 10 Wall Ball Shots															
243	10 Rounds for time: - 5 Clean-and-Jerks - 5 Bar Over Burpees															
	5 Rounds for time of:															

		Day 1			Day 2			Day 3			Day 4			Day 5		
	WORKOUTS	Reps	Time	Weight	Reps	Time	Weight	Reps	Time	Weight	Reps	Time	Weight	Reps	Time	Weight
244	- 10 Overhead Squats															
	- 50 Double-unders															
245	10 Rounds for time:															
	- 100-meter Run															
	- 20 Kettlebell Swings															
	- 10 Pull-Ups															
246	As many reps as possible in 18 minutes:															
	- 80 Double-unders															
	- 10 Wall Ball Shots															
	- 8 Deadlifts															
	- 18 Bar Facing Burpees															
	- 10 Wall Ball Shots															
247	Four parts in 12 minutes every minute on the minute for 3 minutes:															
	-15 Dumbbell Rows															
	- 10 Push-Ups															
	-10 Dumbbell Rows															
	every minute on the minute for 3 minutes:															
	-10 Push-Ups															
	every minute on the minute for 3 minutes:															
	-5 Dumbbell Rows															
	-10 Push-Ups then, as many reps as possible in 3 minutes: Dumbbell Rows															
248	For time:															
	- 10 Kettlebell Swings															
	- 10 Wall Ball Shots															
	- 10 Overhead Squats															
	- 10 Burpees															
	- 10 Lunges															
	- 10 Push Jerks															
	- 10 Knees-to-elbows															
	- 10 Box Jumps															
	- 10 Hang Cleans															
	- 10 Sit-ups															
	- 10 Double-unders															
	- 10 Deadlifts															
249	For time:															
	- 50 Hang Power Snatches															
	- 40 Push Presses															
	- 30 Sumo Deadlift High Pulls															
250	4 Rounds for time of:															
	- 400-meter Row															
	- 10 Deadlifts															
	- 20 Box Jumps															
251	For time:															
	- 20 Alternate Jumping Lunges															
	- 20 Dumbbell Sumo Deadlifts															
	- 20 Dumbbell Push Presses															
	- 15 Alternate Jumping Lunges															
	- 15 Dumbbell Sumo Deadlifts															
	- 15 Dumbbell Push Presses															

		Day 1			Day 2			Day 3			Day 4			Day 5		
	WORKOUTS	Reps	Time	Weight	Reps	Time	Weight	Reps	Time	Weight	Reps	Time	Weight	Reps	Time	Weight
	- 10 Alternate Jumping Lunges															
	- 10 Dumbbell Sumo Deadlifts															
	- 10 Dumbbell Push Presses															
	For time:															
	- 10 Dumbbell Goblet Squats															
252	- 30 Push-Ups															
	- 50 Air Squats															
	- 30 Push-Ups															
	- 10 Dumbbell Goblet Squats															
	For time:															
	- 60-second Max Up-Downs															
253	- 60-second Max Dumbbell Hang Power Cleans															
	- 60-second max Renegade Rows															
	For time:															
254	- 10-9-8-7-6-5-4-3-2-1 Dumbbell Squat Cleans															
	- 11 Burpees															
	5 Rounds for time of:															
255	- 20 Dumbbell Hang Power Cleans															
	- 20 Renegade Row (Alternate arms) with Pushup															
	As many rounds as possible in 20 minutes of:															
256	- 10 Dumbbell Hang Snatches (Alternate arms)															
	- 10 Burpees															
	- 10 Push Jerks															
	For time:															
	- 30 High Knees															
	- 40 Squats															
257	- 50 Jumping Jacks															
	- 60 Reverse Lunges (Alternating Legs)															
	- 70 Burpees															
	- 80 V-ups															
	- 90 Russian Twists															
	For time:															
	- 20 Squats															
	- 20 Sit-ups															
	- 20 Push-Ups															
258	- 20 Front Lunges (Alternating Legs)															
	- 20 Sit-ups															
	- 20 Reverse Lunges (Alternating Legs)															
	- 20 Push ups															
	- 20 Sit-ups															
	- 20 Push ups															
	11 Rounds for time of:															
	- 11 Air Squats															
259	- 11 Front Lunges (Alternating Legs)															
	- 11 Side Leg Swings (Each Leg)															
	- 11 Reverse Lunges (Alternating Legs)															
	- 11 Push-Ups															
	5 Rounds for time of:															

	WORKOUTS	Day 1			Day 2			Day 3			Day 4			Day 5		
		Reps	Time	Weight	Reps	Time	Weight	Reps	Time	Weight	Reps	Time	Weight	Reps	Time	Weight
260	- 20 Crunches - 25 Push-Ups - 30 Jumping Jacks - 35 Air Squats - 45-second Plank															
261	As many rounds as possible in 10 minutes of: - 10 Power Jacks - 10 Mountain Climbers - 10 Curtsy Lunges - 10 Speed skaters															
262	4 Rounds for time of: - 20 Air Squats - 20 Push-Ups - 20 Front Lunges (Alternating Legs) - 1-minute plank - 60 Jumping Jacks															
263	For time: - 20 Air Squats - 20 Second plank - 20 Knee pull-ins - 20 Butt Kicks - 20 Russian Twists - 20 Jumping Jacks															
264	For time: - 5 Tricep Dips - 10 Sit-ups - 15 Push ups - 20 Air Squats - 25 Front Lunges (Alternating Legs) - 30 Jumping Jacks - 25 Second plank - 20 Crunches - 15 Seconds wall Sit - 10 Butt Kicks - 5 Tricep Dips															
265	6 Rounds for time: - 2 Power Snatches - 4 Push Jerks - 6 Overhead Squats - 8 Overhead Walking Lunges															
266	As many reps as possible in 20 minutes: - 20 Wall Ball Shots - 20-Calorie Row															
267	5 Rounds for time of: - 50-ft. Dumbbell Front-rack lunge - 15 Pull-Ups															
268	5 Rounds for time of: - 15 Sit-ups - 30 Squats - 45 Single-unders															

		Day 1			Day 2			Day 3			Day 4			Day 5		
	WORKOUTS	Reps	Time	Weight	Reps	Time	Weight	Reps	Time	Weight	Reps	Time	Weight	Reps	Time	Weight
269	Complete as many rounds as possible in 11 minutes of:															
	- 11 Dumbbell Deadlifts															
	- 7 Burpees															
	- 3 Dumbbell Power Cleans															
270	As many reps as possible in 12 minutes:															
	- 4 Toes-to-Bars															
	- 8 Dumbbell Thrusters															
	- 12 Dumbbell Walking Lunges															
271	As many reps as possible in 20 minutes:															
	- 10 Burpees															
	- 30 Deadlifts															
	- 60 Box Jumps															
	- 70 Sit-ups															
272	5 Rounds for time of:															
	- 25 Kettlebell Swings															
	- 25 GHD Sit-ups															
	- 25 Back Extensions															
	- 25 Knees-to-elbows															
273	5 Rounds for time of:															
	- 500-meter Run															
	- 4 Rope Climbs															
274	Complete as many rounds as possible in 7 minutes of:															
	- 5 Overhead Squats															
	- 5 Box Jumps															
275	21-15-9 Reps for time:															
	- Cleans															
	- Ring Dips															
276	5 Rounds for time of:															
	- 500-meter Run															
	- 20 Overhead Squats															
277	As many reps as possible in 25 minutes:															
	- 5 Deadlifts															
	-13 Push-Ups															
	- 9 Box Jumps															
278	As many reps as possible in 8 minutes:															
	- 1 Pull-up															
	- 2 Push Presses															
	- 2 Pull-Ups															
	- 4 Push Presses continue with this pattern, adding 1 Pull-up and 2 Push Presses each round.															
279	3 Rounds for total reps in 20 minutes:															
	- 1 minute Wall Ball Shots															
	- 1 minute Sumo Deadlift high-pulls															
	- 1 minute Box Jumps															
	- 1 minute Push press															
	- 1 minute Row															
	- 1 minute Rest															

	WORKOUTS	Day 1			Day 2			Day 3			Day 4			Day 5		
		Reps	Time	Weight	Reps	Time	Weight	Reps	Time	Weight	Reps	Time	Weight	Reps	Time	Weight
280	For time: - 50 Wall Ball Shots - 25 Pull-Ups - 50 Sit-ups - 25 Air Squats - 50 Push-Ups - 20-Calorie Air Bike - 50 Kettlebell Swings															
281	Complete as many rounds as possible in 12 minutes of: - 1 Squat Snatch - 3 Clean and Jerks - 30 Double-unders															
282	10 Rounds for time: - 10 Kettlebell Thrusters - 15 Kettlebell sumo Deadlift high-pulls - 10 Burpee Box Jumps - 15 Calorie Assault Air Bike															
283	For time: - 40 Kettlebell Swings - 800-meter Run - 40 Kettlebell Swings															
284	3 Rounds for time: - 15 Dumbbell Deadlifts - 9 Pull-Ups - 3 Curtis P - Rest two minutes 3 Rounds for time: - 20 Dumbbell Overhead Lunge (Alternating lunge) - 10 Toes to Bar - 5 Man Makers finisher 5 minute Cardio of choice															
285	10 Rounds for time: - 10 Mountain Climbers - 10 Air Squats - 10 Hand Release Push-Ups - 10 Box Jump Burpees - 200-meter Run															
286	10 Rounds for time: - 5 Squat Cleans - 10 Burpee Box Jumps															
287	70-40-10 Reps for time: - Burpees - Push-Ups - Sit-ups - Air Squats															
288	As many rounds as possible in 25 minutes of: - 10 Tuck Jumps - 30 Russian Twists - 50 Jumping Jacks - 70 Reverse Lunges (Alternating Legs)															

		Day 1			Day 2			Day 3			Day 4			Day 5		
	WORKOUTS	Reps	Time	Weight	Reps	Time	Weight	Reps	Time	Weight	Reps	Time	Weight	Reps	Time	Weight
	- 90 Burpees															
	- 70 Mountain Climbers															
	- 50 Jumping Jacks															
	- 30 Russian Twists															
	- 10 Tuck Jumps															
289	8 Rounds for time: - 400-meter Run - 20 Back Squats															
290	18-15-12-9-6-3 Reps for time: - Kettlebell Taters - Kettlebell Over Burpees - 50-meter Bear Crawl Shuttles															
291	For time: - 400 Kettlebell Goblet Squats - Perform 10 Kettlebell Russian Twists every time you stop															
292	10-20-30- 40-50- 40-30-20-10 Reps for time: - Air Squats - Russian Kettlebell Swings															
293	21-15-9 Reps for time of: - Dumbbell Ground-to-Overheads - Push-Ups															
294	9-15-21 Reps for time of: - Dumbbell Swings - Push-Ups															
295	For time of 10-20-30 Reps of: - Dumbbell Hang Squat Thrusters - Burpees Over Dumbbell - V-ups															
296	As many rounds as possible in 20 minutes of: - 500-meter Run - 20 Dumbbell Power Cleans															
297	For time: - 50 Burpees - 50 Crunches - 50 Russian Twists - 50 Push-Ups															
298	3 Rounds for time of: - 10 Squats - 10 Push-Ups - 10 Triceps Dips - 10 Steps-ups (Alternating Legs) - 10 Reverse Lunges (Alternating Legs) - 10 Air Squats															
299	7 Rounds for time of: - 20 Russian Twists - 20 Push-Ups - 20 Air Squats															
300	For time: - 500-meter Row - 25 Sit-ups - 750-meter Row - 25 Sit-ups - 1000-meter Row - 25 Sit-ups															

	WORKOUTS	Day 1			Day 2			Day 3			Day 4			Day 5		
		Reps	Time	Weight	Reps	Time	Weight	Reps	Time	Weight	Reps	Time	Weight	Reps	Time	Weight
301	10 Rounds for time of: - 10 Hand Power Snatch - 10 Box Jumps															
302	5 Rounds for time of: - 1-minute Plank hold - 21 Sit-ups															
303	Complete as many rounds as possible in 20 minutes of: - 20 Squats - 40 Single-unders															
304	For time: - 25 Pull-Ups - 50 Deadlifts - 50 Push-Ups - 50 Box Jumps - 50 Floor wipers - 50 Alternating Kettlebell Clean-and-Presses - 3 Rope Climbs - 25 Pull-Ups															
305	For time: - 1500-meter Row then, 5 rounds of: - 10 Bar Muscle-ups - 5 Push Jerks															
306	As many reps as possible in 15 minutes: - 10 Hang Power Snatches - 10 Burpees - 10 Thrusters - 10 Pull-Ups															
307	3 Rounds for time: - 10 Burpees - 10 Thrusters - 10 Burpees - 10 Power Snatches - 10 Burpees - 10 Push Jerks - 10 Burpees - 10 Hang Squat Cleans - 10 Burpees - 10 Overhead Squats															
308	For time: - 25 Walking Lunges - 25 Chest-to-Bar Pull-Ups - 25 Box Jumps - 25 Triple-unders - 25 Back Extensions - 25 Ring Dips - 25 Knees-to-elbows - 25 Wall ball - 25 Sit-ups															
309	For time: - 25 Deadlifts - 25 Ground-to-Overheads - 25 Power Cleans - 25 Burpees															
	As many reps as possible in 20 minutes: - 40 Burpees - 20 Snatches															

	WORKOUTS	Day 1 Reps	Day 1 Time	Day 1 Weight	Day 2 Reps	Day 2 Time	Day 2 Weight	Day 3 Reps	Day 3 Time	Day 3 Weight	Day 4 Reps	Day 4 Time	Day 4 Weight	Day 5 Reps	Day 5 Time	Day 5 Weight
310	- 30 Burpees															
	- 20 Snatches															
	- 20 Burpees															
	- 20 Snatches															
	- 10 Burpees															
311	For time:															
	- 20 Burpees															
	- 20 Sit-ups															
	- 20 Push-Ups															
	- 20 Tuck Jumps															
	- 20 Squats															
	- 20 Jumping Jacks															
	- 20 Lunges															
	- 30 Crunches															
312	21-17-13 Reps for time of:															
	- Push-Ups															
	- Cleans															
313	For time:															
	- 100 Burpee Pull-Ups															
314	Every other minute on the minute for 20 minutes:															
	- 30 Double-unders															
	- max Push-up + renegade Rows															
315	As many reps as possible in 20 minutes:															
	- 10 Deadlifts															
	- 10 Burpee															
	- 10 Kettlebell Swings															
	- 100-meter Run															
316	As many reps as possible in 20 minutes:															
	- 5 Squat Cleans															
	- 5 Push press															
	- 5 Back Squats															
317	4 Rounds for time of:															
	- 250-meter Run															
	- 25 Thrusters															
318	5 Rounds for time:															
	- 10-Calorie Assault Bike															
	- 10 Burpees															
319	3 Rounds for time of:															
	- Run 500-meters															
	- 30 Deadlifts															
320	Complete as many rounds as possible in 10 minutes of:															
	- 5 Power Snatches															
	- 10 Overhead Walking Lunges															
	- 1 Rope climb															
	Complete as many rounds as possible in 15 minutes of:															

		Day 1			Day 2			Day 3			Day 4			Day 5		
	WORKOUTS	Reps	Time	Weight	Reps	Time	Weight	Reps	Time	Weight	Reps	Time	Weight	Reps	Time	Weight
	- 10 Hanging Knee Raises															
321	- 15-Calorie Row															
	- 25 Push-Ups															
	- 15 Box Jumps															
	- 10 Pull-Ups															
	Complete as many rounds as possible in 10 minutes of:															
	- 5 Push press															
322	- 30 Jumping Ropes															
	Rest 2 minutes - complete as many rounds as possible in 10 minutes of:															
	- 5 Hang Power Cleans															
	- 30 Jumping Ropes															
	For time:															
	- 20 Box Jumps															
	- 20 Jumping Pull-Ups															
	- 20 Kettlebell Swings															
	- 20 Walking-Lunge Steps															
323	- 20 Knees-to-elbows															
	- 20 Push Presses															
	- 20 Back Extensions															
	- 20 Wall-Ball Shots															
	- 20 Burpees															
	- 20 Double-unders															
	As many reps as possible in 20 minutes:															
	- 10 Pull-Ups															
	- 10 Push-Ups															
	- 10 Air Squats															
	- 10 Abmat Sit-ups															
	- 10 Kettlebell Swings															
324	- 10-Calorie Row															
	- 10 Toes-to-Bars															
	- 10 Wall Ball Shots															
	- 10 Box Jumps															
	- 10 Alternating Dumbbell Snatches															
	- 10 Burpees															
	- 10 Dumbbell Thrusters															
	For time:															
	- 20 Air Squats															
325	- 20 Snatches															
	- 20 Push-Ups															
	- 20 Thrusters															
	10 Rounds for time:															
	- 6 Wall Ball Shots															
326	- 4 Handstand Push-Ups															
	- 2 Power Clean															
	5 Rounds for time:															
327	- 10 Deadlifts															
	- 10 Hand Power Cleans															
	For time:															
	- 1 Wall Walk															
	- 10 Burpees															
	- 3 Wall Walks															
328	- 20 Burpees															
	- 6 Wall Walks															
	- 30 Burpees															
	- 9 Wall Walks															
	- 40 Burpees															
	5 Rounds of:															
	- 10 Bench Presses															

	WORKOUTS	Day 1			Day 2			Day 3			Day 4			Day 5		
		Reps	Time	Weight	Reps	Time	Weight	Reps	Time	Weight	Reps	Time	Weight	Reps	Time	Weight
329	- 10 Bent Over Rows															
	- 10 Skull Crushers															
	- 10 Bicep Curls															
330	For time:															
	- 10 Overhead Squats															
	- 10 Box Jump-Overs															
	- 10 Thrusters															
	- 10 Power Cleans															
	- 10 Toes-to-Bars															
	- 10 Burpee Muscle-ups															
	- 10 Toes-to-Bars															
	- 10 Power Cleans															
	- 10 Thrusters															
	- 10 Box Jump-Overs															
	- 10 Overhead Squats															
331	21-15-9 Reps for Time:															
	- Dumbbell Thrusters															
	- Pull-Ups															
332	Complete as many rounds as possible in 20 minutes of:															
	- 30-Second Seated Leg Raises															
	- 15 Elevated Push-Ups															
	- 60 Single-unders															
333	10 Rounds for time of:															
	- 8 Ground-to-Overheads															
	- 10 Bar-Facing Burpees															
334	For time:															
	- 500-meter Row															
	- 15 Clean-and-Jerks															
	- 500-meter Row															
	- 25 Burpees															
	- 500-meter Row															
	- 35 Wall Ball Shots															
	- 500-meter Row															
335	5 Rounds of:															
	- 20 Pull-Ups															
	- 30 Push-Ups															
	- 40 Sit-ups															
	- 50 Squats															
336	For time:															
	- 60 Air Squats															
	- 30 Sit-ups															
	- 40 Air Squats															
	- 20 Sit-ups															
	- 20 Air Squats															
	- 10 Sit-ups															
337	10-9-8-7-6-5-4-3-2-1 Reps for time of:															
	- Dumbbell Ground to Overhead															
	- Dumbbell Squats															
338	For time:															
	- 10 Deadlifts															
	- 10 Double Kettlebell Swings															
	- 10 Push-Ups															
	- 10 Clean-and-Jerks															
	- 10 Pull-Ups															
	- 10 Kettlebell Taters															
	- 10 Box Jumps															
	- 10 Wall Climbs															
	- 10 Knee-to-elbows															
	- 10 Double-unders															
339	5 Rounds for time:															
	- 500-meter Run															
	- 15 Overhead Squats															
	- 15 Bar Facing Burpees															

		Day 1			Day 2			Day 3			Day 4			Day 5		
	WORKOUTS	Reps	Time	Weight	Reps	Time	Weight	Reps	Time	Weight	Reps	Time	Weight	Reps	Time	Weight
340	Complete as many reps as possible in 12 minutes of: - Burpees															
341	As many reps as possible in 15 minutes: - 5 Handstand Push-Ups - 10 Pistols (Alternating Legs) - 15 Pull-Ups															
342	Complete as many rounds as possible in 10 minutes of: - 50 Single-unders - 100-m Farmers Carry															
343	5 Rounds for time of: - 3 Power Cleans - 250-meter Run															
344	8 Rounds for time: - 10 Man Makers - 10 Dumbbell Deadlifts - 10 Single-arm Dumbbell Snatches (5 per side) - 10 Single-arm Overhead Lunges (5 per side) - 10 Kettlebell Swings															
345	7 Rounds for time of: - 7 Double Kettlebell Deadlifts - 7 Kettlebell Snatches (Right-Arm) - 7 Kettlebell Snatches (Left-Arm) - 7 meter Bear Crawl Kettlebell Drag (Forward move) - 7 meter Bear Crawl Kettlebell Drag (Backward move)															
346	For time: - 10-9-8-7-6-5-4-3-2-1 Kettlebell Overhead Squat (each arm) - 2-4-6-8-10-12-14-16-18-20 Kettlebell Swings															
347	For time: - 100 Goblet Squats - Every break, perform: - 10 Russian Twists with Kettlebell															
348	For time: - 2000-meter Run - 21 Air Squats - 5 Burpees - 21 Dumbbell Shoulder Presses - 5 Burpees - 21 Dumbbell Lunges - 5 Burpees - 21 Bicep Curls - 5 Burpees - 2000-meter Run															

		Day 1			Day 2			Day 3			Day 4			Day 5		
	WORKOUTS	Reps	Time	Weight	Reps	Time	Weight	Reps	Time	Weight	Reps	Time	Weight	Reps	Time	Weight
	For time for 30-20-15 Reps of:															
349	- Dumbbell Thrusters															
	- Push-Ups															
	For time:															
	- 50 Dumbbell Lunges (Alternate Legs)															
	- 40 Sit-Ups															
	- 30 Burpees															
350	- 20 Hand Release Push-Ups															
	- 10 Dumbbell Deadlifts															
	- 20 Hand Release Push-Ups															
	- 30 Burpees															
	- 40 Sit-Ups															
	- 50 Dumbbell Lunges (Alternate Legs)															
	4 Rounds for time of:															
	- 20 Russian Twists															
	- 20 Crunches															
351	- 20 Jumping Jacks															
	- 20 Mountain Climbers															
	- 20 High Knees															
	For time:															
	- 40 High Knees															
	- 30 Squats															
	- 20 Push-Ups															
352	- 10 Burpees															
	- 20 Front Lunges (Alternating Legs)															
	- 30 Step ups															
	- 40 Jumping Jacks															
	5 Rounds for time of:															
	- 20 High Knees															
	- 20 Mountain Climbers (Alternating Legs)															
	- 20 High Knees															
353	- 20 Climber taps (Alternating Legs)															
	- 20 Flutter Kicks															
	- 20 Scissors															
	- 20 High Knees															
	- 20 Hand Release Push-Ups															
	Complete as many rounds as possible in 20 minutes of:															
	- 5 Jumping Chest-to-Bar Pull-Ups															
354	- 10 Push-Ups															
	- 20 Walking Lunges															
	*after every 3 rounds, 500-meter Run															
	8 Rounds of:															
355	- 2 minute of Rowing Rest 15 seconds															
	- 30-second of Push-Ups Rest 15 seconds															
	4 Rounds for time of:															
356	- 20 Thrusters															
	- 20 Pull-ups															
	As many reps as possible in 25 minutes:															
	- 1 Rope climb															
357	- 6 Pull-Ups															
	- 6 Front Squats															
	- 4 Shoulder-to-Overheads															
	4 Rounds for time of:															
	- 15 Dumbbell Push Jerks															

		Day 1			Day 2			Day 3			Day 4			Day 5		
	WORKOUTS	Reps	Time	Weight	Reps	Time	Weight	Reps	Time	Weight	Reps	Time	Weight	Reps	Time	Weight
358	- 50 Single-unders															
	- 15 Step-ups															
	- 50 Single-unders															
359	5 Rounds for time:															
	- 20 Handstand Push-Ups															
	- 20 Deadlifts															
	- 20 Sit-ups															
	- 20 Double-unders															
360	For time:															
	- 500-m Row															
	- 50 Pull-ups															
	- 10-meter Walking lunge, weight back-racked															
	- 10-meter Walking lunge, weight Front-racked															
	- 10-meter Walking lunge, weight Overhead															
361	5 Rounds for time:															
	- 20 Air Squats															
	- 20 Alternating Lunges															
	- 20 Alternating Split Squat Jumps															
	- 15 Squat Jumps															
362	7 Rounds for time:															
	- 10 Back Squats															
	- 200-meter Row															
363	21-15-9 Reps for time:															
	- Kettlebell Swings															
	- Burpees															
364	4 Rounds for time of:															
	- Run 600 Meters															
	- Rest 2 minutes															
365	4 Rounds for time:															
	- 6 Left-hand Turkish Get-ups															
	- 6 Right-hand Turkish Get-ups															
	- 4 Rope Climbs															
366	As many reps as possible in 20 minutes:															
	- 20-Calorie Ski erg															
	- 20 Sandbag Lunges															
	- 20 Burpee Broad Jumps															
367	Every minute on the minute for 20 minutes:															
	- Odd minutes: 24 Calorie Assault Bike															
	- Even minutes: 18 GHD Sit-ups															
368	5 Rounds for time:															
	- 400-meter Run															
	- 40 Box Jumps															
	- 40 Wall Ball Shots															
369	4 Rounds of:															
	- 5 minutes of Rowing															
	1 minutes of Rest															
370	For time:															
	- 100-Calorie Row															
	- 100-Calorie Ski ERG															

		Day 1			Day 2			Day 3			Day 4			Day 5		
	WORKOUTS	Reps	Time	Weight	Reps	Time	Weight	Reps	Time	Weight	Reps	Time	Weight	Reps	Time	Weight
370	- 100-Calorie Assault Air Bike every 2 minutes, perform:															
	- 7 Burpees															
	5 Rounds for time of:															
371	- 500-meter Row															
	- 5 Thrusters															
	5 Rounds for time:															
372	- 15 Kettlebell Swings															
	- 15 Power Cleans															
	- 15 Box Jumps															
	Complete as many rounds as possible in 15 minutes of:															
373	- 15 Box Jumps															
	- 12 Push Presses															
	- 9 Toes-to-Bars															
	For time:															
	- 350-meter Row															
	- 20 Push Presses															
	- 350-meter Row															
374	- 15 Push Presses															
	- 350-meter Row															
	- 10 Push Presses															
	- 350-meter Row															
	- 5 Push Presses															
	For time:															
	- 500-meter Row															
	- 20 Pull-Ups															
	- 10 Overhead Squats															
375	- 10 Pull-Ups															
	- 20 Overhead Squats															
	- 10 Pull-Ups															
	- 30 Overhead Squats															
	- 500-meter Row															
	As many reps as possible in 20minutes:															
	- 10 Pull-Ups															
	- 10 Push Presses															
376	- 10 Box Jumps															
	- 10 Kettlebell Swings															
	- 10 Toes-to-Bars															
	- 10 Power Cleans															
	- 10 Burpees															
	For time: 10-9-8-7-6-5-4-3-2-1 reps of:															
377	- Hand Release Push-Ups															
	- Air Squats															
	- Sit ups															
	4 Rounds of:															
	- 25 Push-Ups															
378	- 25 Deadlifts															
	- 25 Sit-ups															
	- 50 Single-unders															
	For time:															
379	- 100 Thrusters															
	- 10 Burpees to start and at the top of every minute															

		Day 1			Day 2			Day 3			Day 4			Day 5		
	WORKOUTS	Reps	Time	Weight	Reps	Time	Weight	Reps	Time	Weight	Reps	Time	Weight	Reps	Time	Weight
380	Complete as many rounds as possible in 12 minutes of:															
	- 6 Power Cleans															
	- 12 Hanging Knee-Raises															
381	As many reps as possible in 25 minutes:															
	- 5 Renegade Rows															
	- 10 Burpee Box Jump Over															
	- 15 Abmat Sit ups															
	- 20 Dumbbell Overhead Walking Lunges															
	- 25 Double-unders															
382	Complete as many rounds as possible in 20 minutes of:															
	- 400-meter Run															
	- 10 Pull-Ups															
383	Complete as many rounds as possible in 12 minutes of:															
	- 4 Shoulder Presses															
	- 8 Sumo Deadlift High Pulls															
	- 12 Front Squats															
	- 3000-meter Run															
384	For time:															
	- 10 Handstand Push-Ups															
	- 15 Deadlifts															
	- 25 Box Jumps															
	- 50 Pull-Ups															
	- 100 Wall Ball Shots															
	- 200 Double-unders															
	- 400-meter Run															
385	6 Rounds for time of:															
	- 6 Front Squats															
	- 6 Push-Ups															
386	For time:															
	- 30 Kettlebell Swings															
	- 200-meter Run															
	- 25 Kettlebell Swings															
	- 400-meter Run															
	- 20 Kettlebell Swings															
	- 800-meter Run															
	- 10 Kettlebell Swings															
387	For time:															
	- 50 Power Snatches															
388	For time:															
	- 10 Power Snatches															
	- 10 Box Jump Overs															
	- 10 Thrusters															
	- 10 Power Cleans															
	- 10 Toes-to-Bars															
	- 10 Burpee Muscle-ups															
	- 10 Toes-to-Bars															
	- 10 Power Cleans															
	- 10 Thrusters															
	- 10 Box Jump Overs															
	- 10 Overhead Squats															
	time cap: 15 mins															
389	Complete as many reps as possible in 30 minutes:															
	- 15 Hang Power Cleans															
	- 15 Bar Facing Burpees															
	- 1000-meter Bike															
	- 15 sumo Deadlift high pulls															

		Day 1			Day 2			Day 3			Day 4			Day 5		
	WORKOUTS	Reps	Time	Weight	Reps	Time	Weight	Reps	Time	Weight	Reps	Time	Weight	Reps	Time	Weight
	- 15 strict Ring Dips															
390	11 Rounds for time:															
	- 11 Burpees															
	- 11 Air Squats															
	- 11 Push-Ups															
	- 11 Sit-ups															
391	Every minute on the minute for 25 minutes perform:															
	- 4 Jumping Pull-Ups															
	- 7 Push-Ups															
	- 10 Squats															
392	For time:															
	- 20 Box Jumps															
	- 20 Jumping Pull-Ups															
	- 20 Kettlebell Swings															
	- 20 Lunges															
	- 20 Knees-to-elbows															
	- 20 Push Presses															
	- 20 Back Extensions															
	- 20 Wall Ball Shots															
	- 20 Burpees															
	- 20 Double-unders time cap: 20 minutes															
393	3 Rounds for time of:															
	- 400-meter Run															
	- 15 Ring Rows															
	- 20 Push-Ups															
	- 25 Squats															
394	For time of 9-9-9 Reps of:															
	- Back Squat															
	- Shoulder Press															
	- Deadlift															
395	For time:															
	- 1000-meter Row															
	- 25 Thrusters															
	- 25 Pull-Ups															
	- 1000-meter Row															
396	6 Rounds for time:															
	- 12 Deadlifts															
	- 9 Hang Power Cleans															
	- 6 Push Jerks															
397	As many reps as possible in 20 minutes:															
	- 50 Wall Ball Shots															
	- 50 Double-unders															
	- 40 Box Jumps															
	- 40 Toes-to-Bars															
	- 30 Chest-to-Bar Pull-Ups															
	- 30 Burpees															
	- 20 Power Cleans															
	- 20 Jerks															
	- 10 Power Snatches															
	- 10 Muscle-ups															
398	20 Rounds for time:															
	- 20 Push-Ups															
	- 6 Strict Pull-Ups															
399	Complete as many repetitions as possible in 10 rounds of:															
	- 10 Dumbbell Thrusters															
	- 10 Pull-Ups															
400	Complete as many rounds as possible in 12 minutes of:															
	- 12 Abmat Sit-ups															
	- 12 Walking Lunges															

		Day 1			Day 2			Day 3			Day 4			Day 5		
	WORKOUTS	Reps	Time	Weight	Reps	Time	Weight	Reps	Time	Weight	Reps	Time	Weight	Reps	Time	Weight
	- 20-meter Waiter Walk															
	30-20-10 Reps for time of:															
401	- Row (Calories)															
	- Wall-Ball Shots															
	For time:															
	- 20 Weighted Lunge Steps															
	- 20 Muscle-ups															
	- 20 Push-Ups															
402	- 20 Hang Power Cleans															
	- 20 Box Jumps															
	- 20 Handstand Push-Ups															
	- 20 Front Squats															
403	For time:															
	- 40 Clean-and-Jerks															
	5 Rounds for time:															
	- 15 Kettlebell Swings															
404	- 15 Push-Ups															
	- 15 Burpees															
	- 100-meter Run															
	As many rounds as possible in 15 minutes:															
	- 30-second Kettlebell Swings (Left-Arm)															
	- 30-second Kettlebell Swings (Right-Arm)															
	- 30-second Kettlebell Snatches (Left-Arm)															
405	- 30-second Kettlebell Snatches (Right-Arm)															
	- 30-second Kettlebell Overhead Reverse Lunges (Left-Arm)															
	- 30-second Kettlebell Overhead Reverse Lunges (Right-Arm)															
	- 30 Push-Ups															
	Every minute on the minute:															
406	- Min 1: 10 Kettlebell Swings + 10 Hollow Rocks															
	- Min 2: 10 Kettlebell Goblet Squats + 10 Butterfly Sit Ups															
	10 Rounds for time of:															
	- 10 Dumbbell Goblet Squats															
407	- 10 Dumbbell Power Snatches (Alternate arms)															
	- 10 Dumbbell Overhead Squats (Alternate arms)															
	5 Rounds for time of:															
	- 5 Dumbbell Thrusters															
408	- 5 Dumbbell Sumo Deadlift High Pulls															
	- 5 Dumbbell Hang Cleans															
	- 5 Burpees															
	For time:															
	- 10 Dumbbell Power Snatches (Left-Arm)															
	- 50 Jumping Jacks															
	- 10 Dumbbell Power Snatches (Right-Arm)															
409	- 50 Jumping Jacks															
	- 10 Dumbbell Renegade Rows (Left-Arm)															
	- 50 Jumping Jacks															
	- 10 Dumbbell Renegade Rows (Right-Arm)															
	For time:															

	WORKOUTS	Day 1			Day 2			Day 3			Day 4			Day 5		
		Reps	Time	Weight	Reps	Time	Weight	Reps	Time	Weight	Reps	Time	Weight	Reps	Time	Weight
	- 100 Jumping-jacks															
	- 90 Butt Kicks															
	- 80 V-ups															
	- 70 Inchworms															
410	- 60 Lateral Lunges (Alternating Legs)															
	- 50 Lunges (Alternating Legs)															
	- 40 Burpees															
	- 30 Air Squats															
	- 20 Sit-ups															
	- 10 Push-Ups															
	For time:															
	- 100 Push-Ups															
411	- 100 Sit-ups															
	- 100 Air Squats															
	- 100 Burpees															
	For time:															
	- 50 Jumping Jacks															
	- 100 V-ups															
412	- 100 Squats															
	- 100 Push-Ups															
	- 50 Jumping Jacks															
	As many rounds as possible in 20 minutes of:															
	- 20 Jumping Jacks															
413	- 20 Squats															
	- 20 Burpees															
	- 20 Front Lunges (Alternating Legs)															
	- 20 Push-Ups															
	As many reps as possible in 25 minutes:															
414	- 10 Chest-to-Bar Pull-Ups															
	- 5 Deadlifts															
	- 10 Handstand Push-Ups															
	6 Rounds for time:															
415	- 20 Kettlebell Swings															
	- 500-meter Run															
	3 Rounds for time of:															
	- 250-meter Row															
416	- 250-meter Run															
	- 25 Sit-ups															
	For time:															
	- Muscle Snatch 1-1-1-1 reps															
417	- Power Snatch 1-1-1-1 reps															
	- Squat Snatch 1-1 -1-1 reps															
	As many reps as possible in 25 minutes:															
	2 Rounds of:															
	- 3 Man Makers															
	- 20 Kettlebell Swings															
418	- 100 Single-unders - Rest 1 minutes and proceed in the remaining time with as many reps as possible of:															
	- 500-meter Run															

		Day 1			Day 2			Day 3			Day 4			Day 5		
	WORKOUTS	Reps	Time	Weight	Reps	Time	Weight	Reps	Time	Weight	Reps	Time	Weight	Reps	Time	Weight
	- 30 Wall Ball Shots															
	- 20-Calorie Row															
	- 10 Burpees															
	For time:															
419	- 100 Sandbag Cleans Over the Shoulder every 90 seconds perform															
	- 5 Pull-Ups															
	As many reps as possible in 12 minutes:															
	- 3 Thrusters															
	- 3 Chest-to-Bar Pull-Ups															
	- 6 Thrusters															
420	- 6 Chest-to-Bar Pull-Ups															
	- 9 Thrusters															
	- 9 Chest-to-Bar Pull-Ups if you complete the round of 9, complete a round of 12, then go on to, 15, etc.															
	10 Rounds for time:															
	- 10 Ground-to-Overheads															
	- 10 Bar Facing Burpees															
421	- 10 Shoulder-to-Overheads															
	- 10 Deadlifts															
	- 10 Box Jumps															
	For time:															
	- 20 Knee Raises															
	- 1000-meter Run															
422	- 20 Knee Raises															
	- 1000-meter Run															
	- 20 Knee Raises															
	For time:															
	- 40 Muscle-ups															
423	- 80-calorie Row															
	- 120 Wall-Ball Shots															
	As many reps as possible in 15 minutes:															
	- 10-Calorie Row															
	- 10 Toes-to-Bars															
424	- 10 Wall Ball Shots															
	- 10 Cleans															
	- 10 Muscle-ups															
	As many reps as possible in 15 minutes:															
	- 5 Burpees															
	- 10 Push-Ups															
425	- 15 Air Squats															
	- 6-meter Bear crawl (3 meter there and back)															
	For total reps:															
	- 3 sets of Shoulder Presses, empty Barbell															
	- 3 sets of Pull-Ups															
	- 3 sets of Push Presses, empty Barbell															
426	- 3 sets of Squats, empty Barbell															
	- 3 sets of Pull-Ups															
	- 3 sets of Push Jerks, empty Barbell															
	- 3 sets of Pull-Ups Rest 30 sec. between sets.															
	As many reps as possible in 10 minutes:															
427	- 3 Squat Cleans															
	- 2 Jerks															
	For time:															

		Day 1			Day 2			Day 3			Day 4			Day 5		
	WORKOUTS	Reps	Time	Weight	Reps	Time	Weight	Reps	Time	Weight	Reps	Time	Weight	Reps	Time	Weight
	- 20 Single-Leg Squat, Alternating															
	- 20-yard Handstand Walk															
	- 30 Single-Leg Squat, Alternating															
428	- 30-yard Handstand Walk															
	- 40 Single-Leg Squat, Alternating															
	- 40-yard Handstand Walk															
	- 50 Single-Leg Squat, Alternating															
	- 50-yard Handstand Walk															
	5 Rounds for time:															
	- 20 Pull-Ups															
	- 30 Push-Ups															
429	- 40 Sit-ups															
	- 50 Air Squats															
	1 minutes Rest															
	Complete as much as possible in 15 minutes of:															
	- 1 Jumping Pull-up + 1 Push-Ups															
	- 5 Medicine-ball Cleans															
	- 2 Jumping Pull-up + 2 Push-Ups															
430	- 10 Medicine-ball Cleans															
	- 3 Jumping Pull-up + 3 Push-Ups															
	- 15 Medicine-ball Cleans															
	- 4 Jumping Pull-up + 4 Push-Ups															
	- 20 Medicine-ball Cleans															
	For time:															
	- 30 Pull-Ups															
	- 40 Wall Ball Shots															
431	- 50 Sit-ups															
	- 40 Kettlebell Swings															
	- 30 Burpees															
	For time:															
	- 10 Dumbbell Snatches															
	- 15 Burpee Box Jump Overs															
	- 20 Dumbbell Snatches															
	- 15 Burpee Box Jump Overs															
	- 30 Dumbbell Snatches															
432	- 15 Burpee Box Jump Overs															
	- 40 Dumbbell Snatches															
	- 15 Burpee Box Jump Overs															
	- 50 Dumbbell Snatches															
	- 15 Burpee Box Jump Overs time cap: 25 minutes															
	9-7-5 Reps for time:															
433	- Muscle-ups															
	- Squat Snatches															
	5 Rounds for time:															
	- 3 Rope Climbs															
434	- 11 Toes-to-Bars															
	- 21 Overhead Walking Lunges															
	- 400-meter Run															
	5 Rounds for time of:															
435	- Lunge 50-meters															
	- Run 200-meters															
	For time:															
	- 40 Ring Rows															
436	- 40 Push-Ups															

		Day 1			Day 2			Day 3			Day 4			Day 5		
	WORKOUTS	Reps	Time	Weight	Reps	Time	Weight	Reps	Time	Weight	Reps	Time	Weight	Reps	Time	Weight
	- 40 Sit-ups															
	- 40 Squats															
437	21-15-9 Reps for time:															
	- Handstand Push-Ups															
	- Ring Dips															
	- Push-Ups															
438	3 Rounds for time:															
	- 500-meter Row															
	- 25 Deadlifts															
	- 25 Box Jumps															
439	For time:															
	- 50 Wall Ball Shots															
	- 45 Deadlifts															
	- 40 Hand Release Push-Ups															
	- 35 Box Jumps															
	- 30 Toes-to-Bars															
	- 25 Burpees															
	- 20 Power Cleans															
	- 15 Push Presses															
	- 10 weighted Lunges															
	- 5 Thrusters															
440	For time:															
	- Run 1500-meters Rest 1 minute															
	- Run 1000-meters Rest 1 minute															
	- Run 500-meters															
441	For time:															
	- 40 Wall Ball Shots															
	- 30 Hang Cleans															
	- 40 Pull-Ups															
	- 30 Deadlifts															
	- 40 Push-Ups															
	- 30 Box Jumps															
	- 40 Kettlebell Swings															
	- 30 Toes-to-Bars															
	- 40 Air Squats															
	- 30 Hang Snatches															
	- 40 Double-unders															
	- 30 Sit-ups															
	- 40 Burpees															
442	For time															
	- 25 Deadlifts															
	- 100-meter Run															
	- 25 Kettlebell Swings															
	- 100-meter Run															
	- 25 Overhead Squats															
	- 100-meter Run															
	- 25 Burpees															
	- 100-meter Run															
	- 25 Chest-to-Bar Pull-Ups															
	- 100-meter Run															
	- 25 Box Jumps															
	- 100-meter Run															
	- 25 Dumbbell Squat Cleans															
	- 100-meter Run															

		Day 1			Day 2			Day 3			Day 4			Day 5		
	WORKOUTS	Reps	Time	Weight	Reps	Time	Weight	Reps	Time	Weight	Reps	Time	Weight	Reps	Time	Weight
	<u>For time:</u>															
	- 10 Bar-Facing Burpees															
443	- 20 Thrusters															
	- 25 Bar-Facing Burpees															
	- 30 Thrusters															
	<u>5 Rounds:</u>															
444	- 10 Hang Power Snatches															
	- 10 Push-Ups															
	<u>For time:</u>															
	- 30 Clean-and-Jerks															
445	- 1000-meter Run															
	- 5 Rope Climbs															
	- 1000-meter Run															
	- 50 Burpees															
	<u>As many reps as possible in 20 minutes:</u>															
446	- 5 Dumbbell man Makers															
	- 5 Box Step ups															
	<u>21-15-9 Reps for time of:</u>															
447	- Push-up															
	- Pull-up															
	<u>As many reps as possible in 30 minutes</u>															
	2 rounds of:															
	- 4 Man Makers															
	- 20 Kettlebell Swings															
448	- 80 Single-unders Rest 2 minutes in the remaining time, as many reps as possible of:															
	- 800-meter Run															
	- 30 Wall Ball Shots															
	- 20-Calorie Row															
	- 10 Burpees															
	<u>As many reps as possible in 24 minutes:</u>															
	- 3 Power Cleans															
449	- 6 Push-Ups															
	- 9 Air Squats															
	- 12 Deadlifts															
	<u>27-21-15-9 Reps for time of:</u>															
450	- Squat Cleans															
	- Push-Ups															
	<u>5 Rounds for time of:</u>															
	- 15 Push-Ups															
451	- 15 Ring Dips															
	- 1000-meter Row															
	<u>15-12-9 Reps:</u>															
452	- Clean-and-Jerks															
	<u>As many reps as possible in 12 minutes:</u>															
	- 2-minute Burpees															
453	- 1-minute Rest															
	- 2-minute Jumping Rope															

		Day 1			Day 2			Day 3			Day 4			Day 5		
	WORKOUTS	Reps	Time	Weight	Reps	Time	Weight	Reps	Time	Weight	Reps	Time	Weight	Reps	Time	Weight
	- 1-minute Rest															
	- 2-minute Jumping Jacks															
454	As many reps as possible in 15 minutes:															
	- 8 Power Cleans															
	- 8 Overhead Presses															
	- 10 Push-Ups															
455	For time:															
	- 20 Pull-Ups + 20 Push-Ups															
	- 20-meter Lunge															
	- 200 Single-unders															
	- 10 Pull-Ups + 10 Push-Ups															
	- 20-meter Lunge															
	- 100 Single-unders															
	- 5 Pull-Ups + 5 Push-Ups															
	- 10-meter Lunge															
	- 60 Single-unders															
456	For time:															
	- 21 Dumbbell Thrusters															
	- 400-meter Run															
	- 15 Dumbbell Thrusters															
	- 400-meter Run															
	- 9 Dumbbell Thrusters															
	- 400-meter Run															
457	For time:															
	- 3000 meter Row															
	- 300 Double-unders															
	- 2 mile Run															
458	Complete as many rounds as possible in 20 minutes of:															
	- 5 Power Cleans															
	- 5 Front Squats															
	- 5 Push Presses															
459	As many reps as possible 10:															
	- 3 Hand Power Cleans															
	- 250-meter Row															
460	For time of:															
	- 10 Jumping Jacks															
	- 10-seconds Rest															
	- 20 Jumping Jacks															
	- 10-seconds Rest															
	- 30 Jumping Jacks															
	- 10-seconds Rest															
	- 40 Jumping Jacks															
	- 10-seconds Rest															
461	Every minute on the minute for 15 minutes:															
	- 5 Squats															
	- 5 Hand Power Cleans															
	- 5 Burpees															
	5 Round of:															

		Day 1			Day 2			Day 3			Day 4			Day 5		
	WORKOUTS	Reps	Time	Weight	Reps	Time	Weight	Reps	Time	Weight	Reps	Time	Weight	Reps	Time	Weight
	- 20 Air Squats															
	- 30 second Up and Down Plank															
462	- 20 Kettlebell Snatches (Split between arms)															
	- 30-second Plank															
	- 24 Overhead Dumbbell Lunges															
	- 12 Burpees															
	- 6 Push-Ups															
	<u>3 Rounds for time of:</u>															
	- 60 Lunges (Alternate Legs)															
	- 50 Air Squats															
463	- 40 Sit-ups															
	- 30 Push-Ups															
	- 20 Burpees															
	- 10 Dumbbell Thrusters															
	<u>For time:</u>															
	- 11 Dumbbell Deadlifts															
	- 11 Spider-Man Push-Ups															
	- 10 Dumbbell Deadlifts															
	- 10 Spider-Man Push-Ups															
	- 9 Dumbbell Deadlifts															
	- 9 Diamond Push-Ups															
	- 8 Dumbbell Deadlifts															
	- 8 Spider-Man Push-Ups															
	- 7 Dumbbell Deadlifts															
	- 7 Diamond Push-Ups															
	- 6 Dumbbell Deadlifts															
464	- 6 Spider-Man Push-Ups															
	- 5 Dumbbell Deadlifts															
	- 5 Diamond Push-Ups															
	- 4 Dumbbell Deadlifts															
	- 4 Spider-Man Push-Ups															
	- 3 Dumbbell Deadlifts															
	- 3 Diamond Push-Ups															
	- 2 Dumbbell Deadlifts															
	- 2 Spider-Man Push-Ups															
	- 1 Dumbbell Deadlift															
	- 1 Diamond Push-Up															
	<u>As many arounds as possible in 12 minutes of:</u>															
465	- 3 Deadlifts															
	- 3 Shoulder Presses															
	<u>5 Rounds for time:</u>															
	- 20 Alternating Jumping Lunges															
466	- 20 Russian Kettlebell Swings															
	- 20 Push-Ups															
	<u>For time:</u>															
467	- 200 Kettlebell Russian Swing															
	*Every Break 500-meter Run															
	<u>For time:</u>															
468	- 50-40-30-20-10 of Kettlebell Swings															
	- 50-meters Bear Crawl															
	- 50-meters Reverse Bear Crawl															
	<u>Complete as many rounds as possible in 15 minutes of:</u>															
469	- 15 Box Jumps															

		Day 1			Day 2			Day 3			Day 4			Day 5		
	WORKOUTS	Reps	Time	Weight	Reps	Time	Weight	Reps	Time	Weight	Reps	Time	Weight	Reps	Time	Weight
	- 12 Push Presses															
	- 9 Toes-to-Bar															
	For time:															
	- 2 Rope Climbs															
	- 30 Squats, Alternating															
	- 30 Dumbbell Snatches (Alternating arms)															
	- 2 Rope Climbs															
	- 20 Squats, Alternating															
470	- 20 Dumbbell Snatches (Alternating arms)															
	- 2 Rope climb															
	- 10 Squats, Alternating															
	- 10 Dumbbell Snatches (Alternating arms)															
	- 2 Rope climb															
	- 5 Squats, Alternating															
	- 5 Dumbbell Snatches (Alternating arms)															
	3 Rounds of:															
	- 10 Push-Ups															
471	- 10 Dumbbell Hang Power Cleans															
	- 50 Single Unders															
	3 Rounds of:															
	- 10 Push-Ups															
472	- 10 Dumbbell Shoulder-to-Overheads															
	- 50 Single Unders															
	As many reps as possible in 10 minutes:															
	- 20-meter Dumbbell Walking Lunges															
	- 16 Toe-to-Bars															
473	- 8 Dumbbell Power Cleans															
	Then, 2 rounds of:															
	- 20-meter Dumbbell Walking Lunges															
	- 16 Snatches															
	- 8 Dumbbell Power Cleans															
	3 Rounds for time of:															
474	- 30 Pull-Ups															
	- 300-meter Run															
	10 Rounds of:															
	- 1-minute of Burpees															
475	- 1-minute of Air Squats															
	- 1-minute of Double unders															
	1 minute Rest															
	As many reps as possible in 10 minutes:															
	- 1 Pull-up															
	- 2 Push Presses															
476	- 2 Pull-Ups															
	- 4 Push Presses continue with this pattern, adding 1 Pull-up and 2 Push Presses each round															

		Day 1			Day 2			Day 3			Day 4			Day 5		
	WORKOUTS	Reps	Time	Weight	Reps	Time	Weight	Reps	Time	Weight	Reps	Time	Weight	Reps	Time	Weight
	As many reps as possible in 20 minutes:															
	- 10 Pull-Ups															
	- 20 Push-Ups															
	- 30 Air Squats															
	- 15 Pull-Ups															
	- 30 Push-Ups															
477	- 45 Air Squats															
	- 20 Pull-Ups															
	- 40 Push-Ups															
	- 60 Air Squats															
	- 25 Pull-Ups															
	- 50 Push-Ups															
	- 75 Air Squats															
	For time:															
	- 21 Dumbbell Thrusters															
	- 400-meter Run															
478	- 18 Dumbbell Thrusters															
	- 400-meter Run															
	- 15 Dumbbell Thrusters															
	- 400-meter Run															
	5 Rounds for time of:															
	- 500-meter Run															
479	- 20 Overhead Squats															
	- 20 Sumo Deadlift High Pulls															
	10 Rounds for time:															
480	- 10 Air Squats															
	- 10 Push-Ups															
	- 10 Mountain Climbers (Left+Right=1)															
	- 10 Jumping Jacks															
	For time:															
	- 10 Dumbbell Snatches (Split reps between arms)															
	- 15 Burpee Box Jump-Overs															
	- 20 Dumbbell Snatches (Split reps between arms)															
	- 15 Burpee Box Jump-Overs															
481	- 30 Dumbbell Snatches (Split reps between arms)															
	- 15 Burpee Box Jump-Overs															
	- 40 Dumbbell Snatches (Split reps between arms)															
	- 15 Burpee Box Jump-Overs															
	- 50 Dumbbell Snatches (Split reps between arms)															
	- 15 Burpee Box Jump-Overs															
	For time:															
	- 10 Burpees															
	- 25 Push-Ups															

	WORKOUTS	Day 1			Day 2			Day 3			Day 4			Day 5		
		Reps	Time	Weight	Reps	Time	Weight	Reps	Time	Weight	Reps	Time	Weight	Reps	Time	Weight
482	- 10 Burpees - 25 Push-Ups - 50 Lunges - 10 Burpees - 25 Push-Ups - 50 Lunges - 10 Burpees - 25 Push-Ups - 50 Lunges - 100 Sit-ups - 150 Air Squats															
483	<u>5 Rounds in 20 minutes of:</u> - 1 minute of Rowing - 1 minute of Burpees - 1 minute of Double-unders - 1 minute Rest															
484	<u>For time:</u> - 100 Pull-Ups - 100 Push-Ups - 100 Sit-ups - 100 Air Squats															
485	<u>12-9-6 Reps for time:</u> - Clean and Jerks - Thrusters															
486	<u>As many reps as possible in 20 minutes:</u> - 500-meter Run - 20 Overhead Squats - 20 Back Squats															
487	<u>Complete as many rounds as possible in 20 minutes of:</u> - 50 Double-unders - 15 Toes-to-Bars															
488	<u>For time:</u> - 100 Dumbbell Hang Clean Thrusters - 5 Burpees to start, and at the top of each minute															
489	<u>3 Rounds for time of:</u> - 200-meter Run - 20 Hanging Knee Raises - 200-meter Run															
490	<u>21-7-11 Reps for time:</u> - Burpees - Kettlebell Swings - Double-unders															
491	<u>5 Rounds for time:</u> - 15 Hollow Rocks - 15 V-ups - 15 Tuck ups - 15 second Hollow Hold 1 minute Rest															
492	<u>For time:</u> - 150 Wall Ball Shots															
493	<u>As many reps as possible in 15 minutes:</u> - 7 Pull-Ups - 11 Push-Ups - 15 Air Squats															
	<u>As many reps as possible in 20 minutes:</u> - 1000-meter Run then, 5 rounds of:															

		Day 1			Day 2			Day 3			Day 4			Day 5		
	WORKOUTS	Reps	Time	Weight	Reps	Time	Weight	Reps	Time	Weight	Reps	Time	Weight	Reps	Time	Weight
494	- 30 Air Squats															
	- 20 Push-Ups if you finish, start again on the Run.															
495	Buy in: 15 Devil Presses then, 3 rounds of:															
	- 8 Burpees															
	- 12 Dumbbell Snatches															
	- 16 Toes to Bar cash out: 15 Devil Presses															
496	For time:															
	- 100 Kettlebell Swings															
	- 100 Sit-ups															
	- 100 Air Squats															
	- 100 Push-Ups															
497	For time:															
	- 2000-meter Row															
	- 100 Wall-Ball Shots															
	- 20 Muscle-ups															
498	As many reps as possible in 20 minutes:															
	- 80 Double-unders															
	- 10 Wall Ball Shots															
	- 10 Deadlifts															
	- 10 Bar Facing Burpees															
	- 10 Wall Ball Shots															
499	21-15-9 Reps for time:															
	- Deadlifts															
	- Handstand Push-Ups															
500	5 2-minute rounds of:															
	- 20 Dumbbell Box Step-ups															
	- max reps of Dumbbell Push Presses															
501	30-20-10-5 Reps for time of:															
	- Row (Calories)															
	- Alternating Dumbbell Hang Snatch															
502	7 Rounds for time:															
	- 7 Handstand Push-Ups															
	- 7 Thrusters															
	- 7 Knees-to-elbows															
	- 7 Deadlifts															
	- 7 Burpees															
	- 7 Kettlebell Swings															
	- 7 Pull-Ups															
503	For time:															
	- 15 Muscle-ups															
	- 150 Double-unders															
	- 12 Muscle-ups															
	- 120 Double-unders															
	- 9 Muscle-ups															
	- 90 Double-unders															
504	For time:															
	- 45 Kettlebell Swings															
	- 400-m Run															
	- 35 Kettlebell Swings															
	- 800-m Run															
	- 25 Kettlebell Swings															
	- 1,200-m Run															
	- 15 Kettlebell Swings															

		Day 1			Day 2			Day 3			Day 4			Day 5		
	WORKOUTS	Reps	Time	Weight	Reps	Time	Weight	Reps	Time	Weight	Reps	Time	Weight	Reps	Time	Weight
505	For time: - 50 Dumbbell Snatches - 5 Rope Climbs - 40 Dumbbell Snatches - 4 Rope Climbs - 30 Dumbbell Snatches - 3 Rope Climbs - 20 Dumbbell Snatches - 2 Rope Climbs															
506	For time: - Run 800-meters (or 5 minutes) then - 5 Rounds of: - 10 Push-Ups - 15 Med-ball Cleans - 15 Burpees															
507	3 Rounds for time of: - Run 800-meters - 50 Back Extensions - 50 Sit-ups															
508	As many rounds as possible in 15 minutes of: - 15-Calorie row - 10 Push-Ups															
509	Complete as many rounds as possible in 20 minutes of: - 5 Pull-Ups - 10 Push-Ups - 15 Air Squats															
510	For time: - 30 Alternating Dumbbell Snatches - 30 Air Squats - 30 Deadlifts - 30 Push-Ups - 30 Hang Cleans - 30 Wall Ball Shots - 30 Russian Kettlebell Swings - 30 Box Jump Overs - 30 Shoulder-to-Overheads - 30 Ball slams															
511	3 Rounds for time of: - 400-meter Run - 30 Box Step-ups - 30 Squats															
512	Complete as many rounds as possible in 20 minutes of: - 2 Muscle-ups - 4 Handstand Push-Ups - 8 Kettlebell Swings															
513	12 Rounds for time, starting with 1 and adding an exercise each round of: - 1 Wall Walk - 2 Candlesticks - 3 Burpees - 4 Push-Ups - 5 Walking Lunges - 6 Air Squats - 7 Sit-ups - 8 Jumping Squats - 9 Jumping Lunges - 10 Broad Jumps - 11 Handstand Push-Ups - 12 Pistols															
	3 Rounds for time: - 15-meter Single-arm Dumbbell Overhead Walking Lunges															

	WORKOUTS	Day 1			Day 2			Day 3			Day 4			Day 5		
		Reps	Time	Weight	Reps	Time	Weight	Reps	Time	Weight	Reps	Time	Weight	Reps	Time	Weight
514	- 15 Calorie Assault Bike															
	- 10-meter Dumbbell Overhead Walking Lunges															
	- 8 Toes-to-Bars															
	Complete as many rounds as possible in 20 minutes of:															
515	- 5 Pull-Ups															
	- 10 Push-Ups															
	- 15 Squats															
	As many reps as possible in 25 minutes:															
	- 5 Devil Presses															
516	- 20 Double Dumbbell Front rack reverse Lunges															
	- 25 Calorie Row															
	12 Rounds for time:															
	- 12 Burpees															
517	- 12 Air Squats															
	- 12 Push-Ups															
	- 12 Sit-ups time cap: 25 minutes															
	Complete as many rounds as possible in 20 minutes:															
518	- 15 Sit-ups															
	- 25 Burpees															
	- 35 Wall-Ball Shots															
	10 Rounds for time of:															
	- 10 Kettlebell Russian Swings															
519	- 10 Air Squats															
	- 10 Kettlebell Thrusters (Alternating arms)															
	6 Rounds for time:															
520	- 12 Kettlebell Deadlifts															
	- 9 Kettlebell Cleans (Each arm)															
	-6 Kettlebell Push Jerk (Each arm)															
	For time:															
	- 10-20-30-40-50 reps															
521	- Kettlebell Snatch (Split reps between															
	* After each round															
	10 Burpees Over Kettlebell															
	For time:															
	- 20 Dumbbell Floor Press															
522	- 20 Dumbbell Thrusters															
	- 20 Dumbbell Sumo Squats															
	- 20 Push-Ups															
	As many reps as possible in 10 minutes															
523	- 10 Dumbbell Push-up with Row (Alternate arms)															
	- 10 Dumbbell Snatches															
	- 10 Dumbbell Squats															
	For time:															
	- 50 Dumbbell Strict Presses															
524	- 50 Dumbbell Pull-Overs															
	- 50 Dumbbell Bent Over Rows															
	For time:															
525	- 50 Dumbbell Man-Makers															

		Day 1			Day 2			Day 3			Day 4			Day 5		
	WORKOUTS	Reps	Time	Weight	Reps	Time	Weight	Reps	Time	Weight	Reps	Time	Weight	Reps	Time	Weight
	- 1000-meter Run															
	- 25 Dumbbell Devil Presses															
526	For time:															
	- 1000-meter Run															
	- Then, 3 Rounds for time of:															
	- 8 Dumbbell Burpees to Presses															
	- 100-meter Farmer's Carry															
	- 8 Dual Dumbbell Overhead Reverse Lunge															
	- 100 Air Squats															
	Finally, perform:															
	- 1000-meter Run															
527	Every minute on the minute for 16 minutes:															
	- 40 seconds Plank with Leg lift (Alternating Legs)															
	- 40 seconds Sit-ups															
	- 40 seconds Hand to toe Crunches															
	- 40 seconds Hand-release Push-Ups															
528	For time:															
	- 60 Jumping Jacks															
	- 10 Squats															
	- 10 Push-Ups															
	- 60 Jumping Jacks															
	- 10 Burpees															
	- 10 Lunges (Each Leg)															
	- 60 Jumping Jacks															
	- 10 Inchworms															
	- 10 Mountain Climbers															
	- 60 Jumping Jacks															
529	5 Rounds for time of:															
	- 20 Air Squats															
	- 20 Push-Ups															
	- 20 Jumping Jacks															
530	Every minute of the minute for 20 minutes:															
	- 30-second High Knees															
	- 30-second Mountain Climbers															
	- 30 Reverse Lunges (Alternating Legs)															
	- 30-second Push-Ups															
	- 30-second Air Squats															
	- 30-second Burpees															
531	5 Rounds for time of:															
	- 10 Deadlifts															
	- 10 Burpees															
	Every minute on the minute for 18 minutes of:															
	- Minute 1: 15 Calorie Row															

	WORKOUTS	Day 1 Reps	Day 1 Time	Day 1 Weight	Day 2 Reps	Day 2 Time	Day 2 Weight	Day 3 Reps	Day 3 Time	Day 3 Weight	Day 4 Reps	Day 4 Time	Day 4 Weight	Day 5 Reps	Day 5 Time	Day 5 Weight
532	- Minute 2: Kettlebell Deadlifts															
	- Minute 3: 20 Plate Ground-to-Overheads															
	- Minute 4: Kettlebell Swings															
	- Minute 5: 20 Sit-ups															
	- Minute 6: Kettlebell Thrusters															
	Start again with the exercises															
533	<u>For time: 5-10-15-10-5 Reps of</u>															
	- Clean															
	- Pull-Ups															
534	<u>Complete as many rounds as possible in 10 minutes of:</u>															
	- 10 Dumbbell Hang Power Cleans															
	- 10 Push-Ups															
535	<u>For time:</u>															
	- 70 Sit-ups															
	- 60 Toes-to-Bars															
	- 50 GHD Sit-ups															
	- 40 Pull-Ups															
	- 30 Pull-Ups															
	- 20 Bar Muscle-ups															
536	<u>For time:</u>															
	Round 1:															
	- 1000-meter Row															
	- 1000-meter Assault Air Bike															
	- 200 Single-unders															
	Round 2:															
	- 750-meter Row															
	- 500-meter Assault Air Bike															
	- 150 Single-unders															
	Round 3:															
	- 500-meter Row															
	- 500-meter mile Assault Air Bike															
	- 100 Single-unders															
	round 4:															
	- 250-meter Row															
	- 500-meter Assault Air Bike															
	- 50 Single-unders															
537	<u>6 Rounds for time:</u>															
	- 6 Front Squats															
	- 6 Pull-Ups															
	- 6 Bench Presses															
	- 6 Deadlifts															
	- 6 Barbell Rows															
	- 6 Shoulder-to-Overheads															

		Day 1			Day 2			Day 3			Day 4			Day 5		
	WORKOUTS	Reps	Time	Weight	Reps	Time	Weight	Reps	Time	Weight	Reps	Time	Weight	Reps	Time	Weight
	As many reps as possible in 20 minutes:															
	- 25 Burpees															
	- 200-meter Run															
	- 25 Kettlebell Swings															
538	- 200-meter Run															
	- 25 Pull-Ups															
	- 200-meter Run															
	- 25 Push-Ups															
	- 200-meter Run															
	As many round as possible n 20 minutes of:															
	- 6 Burpees															
539	- 12 Dumbbell Snatches (Alternating arms)															
	- 6 Toes-to-Bars															
	- 6 Goblet Squats															
	As many reps as possible in 24 minutes:															
	- 6 Handstand Push-Ups															
540	- 12 Pull-Ups															
	- 24 Air Squats															
	30 Muscle-ups for time:															
541	if you cannot do the Muscle-ups, do 60 Pull-Ups and 60 Dips															
	As many reps as possible in 15 minutes:															
542	- 20 Wall Ball Shots															
	- 20-Calorie Row															
	21-15-9 Reps for time:															
	- Burpees															
543	- Kettlebell Swings															
	- Double-unders															
	For time:															
	- 20 Thrusters															
	- 200-meter Run															
544	- 20 Air Squats															
	- 400-meter Run															
	- 20 Thrusters															
	- 800-meter Run															
	As many reps as possible in 25 minutes:															
	- 5 Renegade Rows															
	- 10 Burpee Box Jump Over															
545	- 15 Abmat Sit ups															
	- 20 Dual Dumbbell Overhead Walking Lunges															
	- 25 Double-unders															
	6 Rounds for time:															

	WORKOUTS	Day 1 Reps	Day 1 Time	Day 1 Weight	Day 2 Reps	Day 2 Time	Day 2 Weight	Day 3 Reps	Day 3 Time	Day 3 Weight	Day 4 Reps	Day 4 Time	Day 4 Weight	Day 5 Reps	Day 5 Time	Day 5 Weight
546	- 60 Double-unders															
	- 30 Kettlebell Swings															
	- 15 Burpees															
547	Complete as many reps as possible in 5 minutes of:															
	- Shoulder Presses each time you break, perform 50 Single Unders Rest 1 minute then, complete as many reps as possible in 5 minutes of:															
	- Hang Power Cleans each time you break, perform 20 Squats															
548	For time:															
	- 100 Wall-Ball Shots															
549	As many reps as possible in 18 minutes:															
	- 8 Toes-to-Bars															
	- 18 Overhead Squats															
	- 8 Floor Presses															
	- 18 Calorie Bike															
	- 36 Double-unders															
550	As many reps as possible in 21 minutes:															
	- 7 Burpees															
	- 11 Push-Ups															
	- 22 Kettlebell Swings buy-in: 65 Sit-ups															
551	5 Rounds of:															
	- 1 minute of Burpees															
	- 1 minute of Sit-ups Rest 1 minute															
552	As many reps as possible in 20 minutes:															
	- 2 Handstand Push-Ups															
	- 4 Clean and Jerks															
	- 8 Kettlebell Swings															
553	Run for 35 minutes.															
	- Every 5 minutes, stop and perform 15 Burpees															
554	For time:															
	- 50 Air Squats															
	- 50 Jumping Jacks															
	- 50 Push-Ups															
	- 50 Jumping Jacks															
	- 50 Lunges															
	- 50 Jumping Jacks															
	- 50 Burpees															
	- 50 Jumping Jacks															
	- 50 Mountain Climbers															
	- 50 Jumping Jacks															
	- 50 Mountain Climbers															
	- 50 Jumping Jacks															
	- 50 Burpees															
	- 50 Jumping Jacks															
	- 50 Lunges															
	- 50 Jumping Jacks															
	- 50 Push-Ups															
	- 50 Jumping Jacks															
	- 50 Air Squats															
555	For time:															
	- 4-4-4-4-4-4-4 Hang Power Snatch															
556	For time: 3-9-15-21-15-9-3 Reps of															
	- Deadlifts															
	- Box Jumps															
557	For time:															
	- 50 Wall-Ball Shots															
	- 50-Calories Row															

		Day 1			Day 2			Day 3			Day 4			Day 5		
	WORKOUTS	Reps	Time	Weight	Reps	Time	Weight	Reps	Time	Weight	Reps	Time	Weight	Reps	Time	Weight
558	For time: 50-40-30-20-10 reps of															
	- Calorie Row															
	- Burpees															
	- Lunges (Alternating legs)															
559	4 Rounds for time of:															
	- 2 Rope Climbs															
	- 10 Dips															
	- 12 Abmat Sit-ups															
560	For 20 minutes:															
	- 10 Dumbbell Thrusters															
	- 10 Pull-Ups															
561	5 Rounds for time:															
	- 35 Kettlebell Swings															
	- 30 Push-Ups															
	- 25 Pull-Ups															
	- 20 Box Jumps															
	- 1000-meter Run															
562	15-12-9-6-3 Reps for time of:															
	- Power Cleans															
	- Bar-Facing Burpees															
563	As many reps as possible in 18 minutes:															
	- 250-meter Run															
	- 9 Deadlift															
	- 6 Burpee Bar Muscle-ups															
564	8 Rounds for time:															
	- 24 Air Squats															
	- 24 Push-Ups															
	- 24 Walking Lunges															
	- 400-meter Run															
565	As many reps as possible in 10 minutes:															
	- 5 Shoulder-to-Overheads															
	- 10 Deadlifts															
	- 15 Box Jumps															
566	As many reps as possible in 15 minutes:															
	- 30 Double-unders															
	- 15 Power Snatches															
567	5 Rounds for time:															
	- 15 Deadlifts															
	- 10 Hang Power Cleans															
	- 5 Push Jerks															
568	Complete as many rounds as possible in 7 minutes of:															
	- 50 Double-unders															
	- 10 Overhead Squats															
569	For time:															
	- 24 Back Squats															
	- 8 Rope Climbs															
	- 15 Back Squats															
	- 5 Rope Climbs															
	- 12 Back Squats															
	- 4 Rope Climbs															
570	As many reps as possible in 20 minutes:															
	- 10 Push Presses															
	- 10 Box Jumps															
	- 10 Kettlebell Swings															
	As many reps as possible in 25 minutes:															
	- 10 Pull-Ups															
	- 20 Push-Ups															
	- 30 Air Squats															
	- 15 Pull-Ups															
	- 30 Push-Ups															
	- 45 Air Squats															
	- 20 Pull-Ups															

	WORKOUTS	Day 1 Reps	Day 1 Time	Day 1 Weight	Day 2 Reps	Day 2 Time	Day 2 Weight	Day 3 Reps	Day 3 Time	Day 3 Weight	Day 4 Reps	Day 4 Time	Day 4 Weight	Day 5 Reps	Day 5 Time	Day 5 Weight
571	- 40 Push-Ups - 60 Air Squats - 25 Pull-Ups - 50 Push-Ups - 75 Air Squats - 30 Pull-Ups - 60 Push-Ups - 90 Air Squats															
572	As many reps as possible in 15 minutes: - 10 Sit-ups - 5 Walkouts to Push-Ups - every 2 minutes, complete: - 15 Air Squats															
573	Complete as many rounds as possible in 15 minutes of: - 5 Pull-Ups - 10 Push-Ups - 15 Med-ball Cleans															
574	3 Rounds for time of: - 15 Hand Power Clean - 15 Burpees															
575	As many reps as possible in 21 minutes: - 3 Overhead Squats - 6 Overhead Lunges - 9 Power Snatches - 12 Push-Ups - 15 Calorie Assault Air Bike															
576	10 Rounds for time of: - 20 Air Squats - 3 Power Snatches															
577	As many round as possible in 15 minutes of: - 5 Shoulder-to-Overheads - 10 Burpees - 15 Deadlifts															
578	As many reps as possible in 12 minutes: - 7 Power Cleans - 21 Sit-ups - 11 Pull-Ups - 21 Wall Ball Shots															
579	Complete as many rounds as possible in 15 minutes of: - 12 Burpees - 12 Back Squats															
580	As many rounds as possible in 20 minutes of: - 6 Toes-to-Bars - 9 Dumbbell Hang Clean-and-Jerks - 12 Calorie Row															
581	Complete as many rounds as possible in 12 minutes of: - 3 Ring Rows - 6 Push-Ups - 9 Squats															
582	As many reps as possible in 11 minutes: - 1 Rope climb - 3 Squat Snatches															

		Day 1			Day 2			Day 3			Day 4			Day 5		
	WORKOUTS	Reps	Time	Weight	Reps	Time	Weight	Reps	Time	Weight	Reps	Time	Weight	Reps	Time	Weight
	- 2 Rope Climbs															
	- 4 Squat Snatches continue with this pattern, adding 1 rep to each exercise															
583	21-15-9 Reps for time of:															
	- Snatches															
	- Chest-to-Bar Pull-Ups															
584	As many reps as possible in 15 minutes:															
	- 30 Double-unders															
	- 15 Power Snatches															
585	As many reps as possible in 12 minutes:															
	- 9 Thrusters															
	- 21 Burpees															
	- 15 Kettlebell Swings															
	- 250-meter Row															
586	For time:															
	- 20 Pull-Ups															
	- 50 Deadlifts															
	- 50 Push-Ups															
	- 50 Box Jumps															
	- 50 Floor wipers (one count)															
	- 50 Kettlebell Clean-and-Presses															
	- 20 Pull-Ups															
587	21-18-15-12-9-6-3 Reps for time of:															
	- Front Squats															
	- GHD Sit-ups															
588	For time:															
	- 10 Bench Presses															
	- 10 Power Cleans															
	- 100-meter Run															
	- 8 Bench Presses															
	- 8 Power Cleans															
	- 100-meter Run															
	- 6 Bench Presses															
	- 6 Power Cleans															
	- 100-meter Run															
	- 4 Bench Presses															
	- 4 Power Cleans															
	- 100-meter Run															
	- 2 Bench Presses															
	- 2 Power Cleans															
	- 100-meter Run															
589	As many reps as possible in 13 minutes:															
	- 12 Box Jumps															
	- 6 Thrusters															
	- 6 Bar Facing Burpees															
590	Three 3-minute rounds of:															
	- 100-m Farmers Carry then as many reps as possible of:															
	- 3 Burpees															
	- 7 Kettlebell Swings - Rest 1 minutes between rounds															

	WORKOUTS	Day 1			Day 2			Day 3			Day 4			Day 5		
		Reps	Time	Weight	Reps	Time	Weight	Reps	Time	Weight	Reps	Time	Weight	Reps	Time	Weight
	4 Rounds for time of:															
591	- 400-meter Run															
	- 1-minute Plank hold															
	As many reps as possible in 15 minutes:															
592	- 5 Muscle-ups															
	- 50 Wall Ball Shots															
	- 100 Double-unders															
	For time:															
	- 20 Turkish Get-Ups (Right Arm)															
	- 50 Kettlebell Swings															
593	- 20 Overhead Squats (Left Arm)															
	- 50 Kettlebell Swings															
	- 20 Overhead Squats (Right Arm)															
	- 50 Kettlebell Swings															
	- 20 Turkish Get-Ups (Left Arm)															
	For time:															
	- 100 Kettlebell Swings															
594	- 100 Air Squats															
	- 100 Push-Ups															
	- 100 Sit-Ups															
	For time:															
	- 10 Kettlebell Turkish Get-Ups (Split reps between arms)															
	- 40 Kettlebell Sumo Deadlift High-Pulls															
	- 40 Kettlebell Cleans (Split reps between arms)															
595	- 40 Kettlebell Jerks (Split reps between arms)															
	- 100-meter Kettlebell Waiter Carry															
	- 40 Kettlebell Figure 8 through Legs															
	- 40 American Kettlebell Swings															
	- 40 Kettlebell Deadlifts															
	For time:															
	- 50 Air Squats															
	- 26 Kettlebell Sit-Ups															
	- 26 American Kettlebell Swings (Split reps between arms)															
	- 26 Kettlebell Goblet Squats															
596	- 50-meter Kettlebell Lunges															
	- 26 Kettlebell Bent Over Rows (Split reps between arms)															
	- 26 American Kettlebell Swings (Split reps between arms)															
	- 26 Kettlebell Snatches (Split reps between arms)															
	For time:															
	- 500-Meter Run															
	- 25 Dumbbell Clean and Presses															
597	- 500-Meter Run															
	- 25 Dumbbell Burpees and Presses															
	- 500-Meter Run															
	- 25 Dumbbell Thrusters															
	- 500-Meter Run															
	5 Rounds for time of:															
598	- 5 Dumbbell Man-Makers															
	- 10 Dumbbell Lunges (Alternate Legs)															
	- 15 Burpees															
	For time:															
	- 500-Meter Run															
	- 25 Dumbbell Deadlifts															

		Day 1			Day 2			Day 3			Day 4			Day 5		
	WORKOUTS	Reps	Time	Weight	Reps	Time	Weight	Reps	Time	Weight	Reps	Time	Weight	Reps	Time	Weight
	- 25 Burpees Over Dumbbells															
599	- 1000-Meter Run															
	- 25 Dumbbell Deadlifts															
	- 25 Burpees Over Dumbbells															
	- 500-Meter Run															
	<u>5 Rounds for time of:</u>															
	- 10 Dumbbell Hang Snatches (Alternating arms)															
600	- 15 Sit-Ups															
	- 20 Dumbbell Lunges (Alternating Legs)															
	- 25 Burpees															
	<u>3 Rounds for time of:</u>															
	- 3 minute Marching in place															
	- 20 Tricep Dips															
601	- 20 Crunches															
	- 20 Hand Release Push-Ups															
	- 20 Lunges (Alternating Legs)															
	<u>4 Rounds for time of:</u>															
	- 10 Push-Ups															
602	- 20 Burpees															
	- 40 Jumping Jacks															
	<u>Every minute on the minute for 20 minutes:</u>															
603	- 5 Burpees															
	- 5 Push-Ups															
	- 5 Air Squats															
	<u>5 Rounds for time of:</u>															
	- 20 Triangle Push-Ups															
	- 20 Air punches															
604	- 20 Crunches															
	- 20 Triangle Push-Ups															
	- 20 Air punches (Alternating arms)															
	- 20 Crunches															
	<u>3 Rounds for time of:</u>															
	- 30 Push-Ups															
605	- 30-second Jump Squats															
	- 30 Push-Ups															
	- 30-seconds Jump Squats															
	<u>As many reps as possible in 15 minutes:</u>															
606	- 10 Toes-to-Bars															
	- 10 Sumo Deadlift High-pulls															
	- 10 Push Presses															
	<u>15 Rounds for time:</u>															
	- 15 Kettlebell Swings															
607	- 10 Goblet Squats															
	- 5 Push-Ups															
	<u>For time:</u>															
	- 20 Jumping Bar Muscle-ups															
	- 5 Overhead Squats															
608	- 10 Jumping Bar Muscle-ups															
	- 10 Overhead Squats															
	- 5 Jumping Bar Muscle-ups															
	- 20 Overhead Squats															
	<u>As many reps as possible in 22 minutes:</u>															
	- 20 Wall Ball Shots															
	- 5 Power Snatches															
609	- 20 Box Jumps															
	- 5 Push Presses															

		Day 1			Day 2			Day 3			Day 4			Day 5		
	WORKOUTS	Reps	Time	Weight	Reps	Time	Weight	Reps	Time	Weight	Reps	Time	Weight	Reps	Time	Weight
	- 20-Calorie Row															
	7 Rounds for time:															
	- 7 Push-Ups															
	- 7 GHD Sit-ups															
	- 7 Air Squats															
610	- 7 Pull-Ups															
	- 7 Deadlifts															
	- 7 Hang Power Cleans															
	- 7 Shoulder-to-Overheads															
	- 7 Calorie Row															
	21-15-9 Reps for time:															
611	- Thrusters															
	- Pull-Ups															
	As many reps as possible in 20 minutes:															
	- 5 Pull-Ups															
612	- 10 Push-Ups															
	- 15 Squats															
	- 5 Pull-Ups															
	- 10 Thrusters															
	For time:															
	- 5 sets of: 4 Pull-ups + 4 Push-Ups															
613	- 50 Squats															
	- 5 sets of: 4 Pull-Ups + 4 Push-Ups															
	- 50-Calorie Row															
	For time:															
614	- 1-3-6-9-15-21 Wall Walks															
	- 10-30-60-90-150-210 Double-unders time cap: 16 minutes															
	As many reps as possible in 17 minutes:															
615	- 17 Calorie Assault Air Bike															
	- 17 Kettlebell Swings															
	- 17 Abmat Sit-ups															
	10 Rounds for time of:															
616	- 15 GHD Sit-ups															
	- 10 Thrusters															
	3 Rounds for time of:															
	- 500 meter Run															
617	- 12 Pull-Ups															
	- 21 Kettlebell Swings															
	5 Rounds for time:															
	- 30 Double-unders															
618	- 20 Knees-to-elbows															
	- 10 Handstand Push-Ups															
	50 Rounds for time:															
	- 1 Burpee															
	- 1 Push-up															
619	- 1 Jumping-jack															
	- 1 Sit-up															
	- 1 Air squat															
	6 Rounds for time of:															
	- 12-Calorie Row															
620	- 9 Hang Power Snatches															
	- 6 Burpees															

	WORKOUTS	Day 1			Day 2			Day 3			Day 4			Day 5		
		Reps	Time	Weight	Reps	Time	Weight	Reps	Time	Weight	Reps	Time	Weight	Reps	Time	Weight
621	As many rounds as possible in 18 minutes:															
	- 18 Kettlebell Snatches															
	- 9 Dumbbell Thrusters															
	- 18 Chest-to-Bar Pull-Ups															
	- 9 Devil Presses															
622	6 Rounds for time:															
	- 6 Power Cleans															
	- 12 Front Squats															
	- 6 Jerks															
	- 24 Pull-Ups															
	- 60-second Rest															
623	As many reps as possible in 10 minutes:															
	- 10 Power Cleans															
	- 10 Burpees Over the Bar															
	- 20 Deadlifts															
	- 20 Pull-Ups															
624	For time:															
	- 500-meter Row															
	- 40 Air Squats															
	- 30 Sit-ups															
	- 20 Push-Ups															
	- 10 Pull-Ups															
625	For time: buy-in:															
	- 250-meter Run then, 5 rounds of:															
	- 10 Air Squats															
	- 10 Sit-ups															
	- 10 Burpees															
	cash-out:															
	- 250-meter Run															
626	10 Rounds for time:															
	- 10-meter Handstand Walk															
	- 5 Snatches															
	- 7 Ring Muscle-ups															
627	For time:															
	- 3 Clean-and-Jerks															
	- 3 Toes-to-Bars															
	- 6 Clean-and-Jerks															
	- 6 Toes-to-Bars															
	- 9 Clean-and-Jerks															
	- 9 Toes-to-Bars															
	- 12 Clean-and-Jerks															
	- 12 Toes-to-Bars															
628	20 Minute as many reps as possible:															
	- 14 V-ups															
	- 7 Burpees															
	- 14 Plank Shoulder Taps															
	- 7 Burpees															
	- 14 Windshield wipers															

		Day 1			Day 2			Day 3			Day 4			Day 5		
	WORKOUTS	Reps	Time	Weight	Reps	Time	Weight	Reps	Time	Weight	Reps	Time	Weight	Reps	Time	Weight
	- 7 Burpees															
629	For time:															
	- 50 Deadlifts															
	- 50 Power Clean															
	- 50 Ground-to-Overhead															
	- 50 Burpees															
630	As many reps as possible in 15 minutes:															
	- 200-meter Run															
	- 100 Double-unders															
	- 30 Burpees															
	- 3 Rope Climbs															
631	For time: 20-16-12-8-4 reps of															
	- Bench Presses															
	- Calorie Row															
632	As many reps as possible 15 minutes:															
	- 3 Deadlifts															
	- 6 Hand Power Cleans															
	- 9 Bar Facing Burpees															
633	Complete as many reps as possible in 15 minutes of:															
	- Run 200-meters															
	- 15 Ring Rows															
634	For time:															
	- 10 Thrusters															
	- 10 Bar-Facing Burpees															
	- 20 Thrusters															
	- 10 Bar-Facing Burpees															
	- 30 Thrusters															
	- 10 Bar-Facing Burpees															
635	3 Rounds for total reps in 18 minutes:															
	- 1 minute Burpees															
	- 1 minute Power Snatches															
	- 1 minute Box Jumps															
	- 1 minute Thrusters															
	- 1 minute Chest-to-Bar Pull-Ups															
	- 1 minute Rest															
636	5 Rounds of:															
	- 5 Burpees															
	- 20 Squats															
	- 5 Burpees															
	- 10 Push ups															
	- 5 Burpees															
	- 20 Lunges															
	- 5 Burpees															

	WORKOUTS	Day 1			Day 2			Day 3			Day 4			Day 5		
		Reps	Time	Weight	Reps	Time	Weight	Reps	Time	Weight	Reps	Time	Weight	Reps	Time	Weight
	- 10 V-ups															
637	For time: - 20 Burpees - 250-meter Run - 20 Push-Ups - 250-meter Run - 20 Walking Lunges - 250-meter Run - 20 Air Squats - 250-meter Run - 20 Walking Lunges - 250-meter Run - 20 Push-Ups - 250-meter Run - 20 Burpees															
638	10 Rounds for time: - 5 Devil Presses - 15 Dumbbell Lunges (Alternating legs) - 25 Air Squats															
639	For time: - 50 Power Snatches															
640	As many reps as possible in 25 minutes: - 10 Man Makers - 10 Burpees - 250-meter Run - 10 Air Squats - 10 Handstand Push-Ups															
641	7 Rounds for time: - 10 Push-Ups - 10 Air Squats - Run 200m															
642	Complete as many rounds as possible in 12 minutes of: - 3 Burpee Box Jump-Overs - 3 Deadlifts - 6 Burpee Box Jump-Overs - 6 Hand Power Cleans - 9 Burpee Box Jump-Overs - 9 Push-Ups															
643	5 Rounds for time: - 1 Deadlift - 2 Muscle-ups - 3 Squat Cleans - 4 Handstand Push ups															
644	4 Rounds for time: - 10 Push-Ups - 10 Sit-ups - 10 Box Jumps - 10 Kettlebell Swings - 10 Push Presses - 10 Walking Lunges (each Leg) - 10 Mountain Climbers - 10 Knees-to-elbows - 10 Pull-Ups - 10 Parallel Bar Dips - 10 Air Squats - 10 Back Extensions - 10 Burpees															
645	10 Rounds for time of: - 100-m Sprint - 5 Burpees															

	WORKOUTS	Day 1			Day 2			Day 3			Day 4			Day 5		
		Reps	Time	Weight	Reps	Time	Weight	Reps	Time	Weight	Reps	Time	Weight	Reps	Time	Weight
645	- 20 Sit-ups															
	- 15 Push-Ups															
	- 100-m Sprint Rest 1 minute															
646	As many reps as possible in 20 minutes:															
	- 20 Air Squats															
	- 20 Push-Ups															
	- 20 Kettlebell Swings															
	- 20 Jumping Lunges															
	- 20 Sit-ups															
	- 20 Box Jumps															
647	For time:															
	- 15 Toes-to-Bars															
	- 25-Calorie Row															
	- 50 Push-Ups															
	- 25 Box Jumps															
	- 15 Pull-Ups															
648	10 Rounds for time:															
	- 4 Snatches															
	- 4 Bar Over Burpees															
649	For time:															
	- 10 Push-Ups															
	- 30 Kettlebell Swings															
	- 9 Push-Ups															
	- 30 Kettlebell Swings															
	- 8 Push-Ups															
	- 30 Kettlebell Swings															
	- 7 Push-Ups															
	- 30 Kettlebell Swings															
	- 6 Push-Ups															
	- 30 Kettlebell Swings															
650	3 Rounds for time:															
	- 50-meter Farmer's Carry															
	- 25-meter Walking Lunges															
	- 25 Kettlebell Swings															
	- 25 Goblet Squats															
651	20 Rounds for time of:															
	- 6 Kettlebell Swing															
	- 8 Kettlebell Clean and Push Jerk (Split reps between arms)															
	- 10 Burpees															
	- 12 Kettlebell Russian Swings															
652	5 Rounds for time:															
	- 500-meter Run															
	- 50 Russian Kettlebell Swings															
	- 25 Air Squats															
653	10-8-6-4-2-1 Reps for time:															
	- Burpees															
	- Kettlebell Thrusters (Slit reps between arms)															
	- Burpees															
	- Kettlebell Sumo Deadlift High-Pulls															
	- Burpees															
	- Kettlebell Swings															
	8 Rounds for time:															

	WORKOUTS	Day 1			Day 2			Day 3			Day 4			Day 5		
		Reps	Time	Weight	Reps	Time	Weight	Reps	Time	Weight	Reps	Time	Weight	Reps	Time	Weight
654	- 8 Kettlebell Clean (Split reps between arms)															
	- 8 Burpees															
	- 10 Air Squats															
	- 10 Dumbbell Thrusters															
	- 12 Push-Ups															
	- 12 Burpees															
	- 24 Air Squats															
655	3 Rounds for time of:															
	- 1000-Meter Run															
	- 25 Dumbbell Squat Cleans															
	- 25 Burpees															
	- 25 Push-Ups															
656	10 Rounds for time of:															
	- 10 Dumbbell Hang Clean-and-Jerks (Alternate arms)															
	- 10 Dumbbell Hang Squat Cleans															
657	11 Rounds for time of:															
	- 250-meter Runs															
	- 11 Dumbbell Burpee Deadlifts															
658	21-15-9 Reps for time of:															
	- Dumbbell Thrusters															
	- Air Squats															
	- Burpees															
659	5 Rounds for time of:															
	- 15 Dumbbell Deadlifts															
	- 30 Sit-ups															
	- 15 Dumbbell Shoulder Presses															
	- 15 Dumbbell Squat Cleans															
660	For time:															
	- 10 Hand Release Push-Ups															
	- 20 Tricep Dips															
	- 30 V-ups															
	- 40 Bicycle Crunches															
661	3 Rounds for time of:															
	- 1 minute: High Knees															
	- 1 minute: Jumping Jacks															
	- 1 minute: Front Kicks															
	- 1 minute: Push-Ups															
	- 1 minute: Jumping Jacks															
	- 1 minute: Run in place															
662	Every minute on the minute for 16 minutes:															
	- 4 Burpees															
	- 4 Push-Ups															
663	For time:															
	- 10 Push-Ups															
	- 20 Burpees															
	- 30 Mountain Climbers															
	- 40 Squats															
	- 50 Jumping Jacks															
664	4 Rounds for time of:															
	- 24 Push-Ups															
	- 24 Squats															
	- 24 Burpees															

		Day 1			Day 2			Day 3			Day 4			Day 5		
	WORKOUTS	Reps	Time	Weight	Reps	Time	Weight	Reps	Time	Weight	Reps	Time	Weight	Reps	Time	Weight
	- 24 Pistol Squats															
665	For time: - 1 minute plank - 50 Sit-ups - 50 Russian Twists - 50 Burpees - 50 Inchworms - 50 Push-Ups															
666	5 Rounds for time: - 250-meter Run - 40 Walking Lunges - 30 Sit-Ups - 20 Push-Ups - 10 Kettlebell Swings - 5 Burpees Over Kettlebell															
667	For time: - 300 Kettlebell Swings *Every minute on the minute: 5 Burpees starting at 01:00															
668	20-16-12-8-4 Reps for time: - Kettlebell Cleans (Alternating arms) - Hand Release Push-Ups - Burpees															
669	For time: - 200 Russian Kettlebell Swings - 100 American Kettlebell Swings - Perform the following every time you put the Kettlebell down: - 15 Air Squats - 10 Push-Ups - 5 Burpees															
670	As many rounds as possible in 20 minutes: - 30 Double-unders - 15 Power Snatches															
671	30 Rounds for time of: - 5 Wall Ball Shots - 3 Push-Ups - 1 Power Clean															
672	As many rounds as possible in 21 minutes: - 30 Calorie Row - 20 Burpees Over Rower - 10 Power Cleans															
673	5 Rounds for time: - 600 meter Run - 30 Kettlebell Swings															

		Day 1			Day 2			Day 3			Day 4			Day 5		
	WORKOUTS	Reps	Time	Weight	Reps	Time	Weight	Reps	Time	Weight	Reps	Time	Weight	Reps	Time	Weight
	- 15 Pull-Ups															
	For time:															
	- Row 1000-meters															
	- 50 Dumbbell Squat Snatches (Alternating arms)															
674	- Row 750-meters															
	- 35 Dumbbell Squat Snatches (Alternating arms)															
	- Row 500-meters															
	- 20 Dumbbell Squat Snatches (Alternating arms)															
	3 Rounds for time of:															
675	- 30 Sit-ups															
	- 500-meter Run															
	30-20-10 Reps for time of:															
676	- Toes-to-Bars															
	- Kettlebell Walking Lunges															
	For time:															
677	- 30 Snatches															
	2 Rounds for time:															
	- 25 Deadlifts															
	- 25 Box Jumps															
	- 25 Wall Ball Shots															
678	- 25 Bench press															
	- 25 Box Jumps															
	- 25 Wall Ball Shots															
	- 25 Cleans															
	As many reps as possible in 30 minutes:															
	- 30 Air Squats															
	- 20 Box Jumps															
679	- 30 meter Walking Lunges															
	- 20 Hand Release Push-Ups															
	- 30 Burpees															
	- 50-meter Run															
	As many reps as possible in 20 minutes:															
	- 5 Pull-Ups															
680	- 10 Push-Ups															
	- 15 Air Squats															
	For time:															
	- 20 Hanging Knee Raises															
	- 20 Single-arm Dumbbell Snatches															
681	- 20 Dumbbell Box step-Overs															
	- 20 Single-arm Dumbbell Snatches															
	- 20 Hanging Knee Raises															
	4 Rounds For Time:															
	- 4 Jerks															
682	- 10 Toes-to-Bars															
	- 4 Jerks															
	- 10 Kettlebell Swings															

		Day 1			Day 2			Day 3			Day 4			Day 5		
	WORKOUTS	Reps	Time	Weight	Reps	Time	Weight	Reps	Time	Weight	Reps	Time	Weight	Reps	Time	Weight
683	For time: - 1000-meter Run - 2000-meter Row - 1000-meter Run															
684	4 Rounds for time of: - 500-meter Run - 25 Back Squats															
685	As many reps as possible in 15 minutes: - 5 Handstand Push-Ups - 10 Pull-Ups - 15 Air Squats															
686	9-6-3 Reps for time of: - Snatch - Burpee Box Step-Over															
687	As many reps as possible in 10 minutes: - 10 Snatches - 10 Snatches (increased weight) - 10 Snatches (increased weight)															
688	3 Rounds for time: - 400-meter Run - 16 Bench Presses - 16 Wall Ball Shots - 16 Shoulder-to-Overheads - 16 GHD Sit-ups															
689	10 Rounds for time: - 10 Thrusters - 35 Double-unders time cap: 40 minutes															
690	For time: - 2 minute Elbow plank - 13 Burpees - 18 Kettlebell Swings - 31 Push-Ups - 53 Goblet Squats - 53 Burpees - 31 Kettlebell Swings - 18 Push-Ups - 13 Goblet Squats - 2 minute Wall Sit															
691	As many reps as possible in 22 minutes: - 6 Dumbbell Snatches (Alternating arms) - 6 Man Makers - 6 Burpees - 6 Single Dumbbell Front Squats															
692	For time: - 1000 Box Step-ups															

		Day 1			Day 2			Day 3			Day 4			Day 5		
	WORKOUTS	Reps	Time	Weight	Reps	Time	Weight	Reps	Time	Weight	Reps	Time	Weight	Reps	Time	Weight
693	Complete as many rounds in 12 minutes of: - 6 Front Squats - 12 Chest-to-Bar Pull-Ups - 24 Double-unders															
694	3 Rounds for time: - 12 Deadlifts - 9 Hang Power Cleans - 6 Bar Facing Burpees															
695	5 Rounds for time of: - 20 Power Snatches - 50 Double-unders															
696	3 Rounds for time: - 50 Air Squats - 5 Muscle-ups - 10 Hang Power Cleans															
697	4 Rounds for time: - 20 Kettlebell Ground-to-Overheads - 20 Kettlebell Front Squats - 20 Kettlebell Push-Ups (Alternating arms) - 400-meter Kettlebell Run															
698	6 Rounds for time of: - 30 Squats - 20 Power Cleans - 10 Strict Pull-Ups - Run 500-meters															
699	5 Rounds for time: - 400-meter Run - 30 Back Squats															
700	As many rounds as possible in 10 minutes of: - 3 Clean-and-Jerks - 3 Toes-to-Bars - 6 Clean-and-Jerks - 6 Toes-to-Bars - 9 Clean-and-Jerks - 9 Toes-to-Bars - 12 Clean-and-Jerks - 12 Toes-to-Bars If you complete the round of 12, go on to 15, 18, etc.															
701	As many reps as possible in 15 minutes: - 25 Burpees - 250-meter Run - 25 Kettlebell Swings - 250-meter Run - 25 Pull-Ups															

		Day 1			Day 2			Day 3			Day 4			Day 5		
	WORKOUTS	Reps	Time	Weight	Reps	Time	Weight	Reps	Time	Weight	Reps	Time	Weight	Reps	Time	Weight
	- 250-meter Run															
	- 25 Push-Ups															
	- 250-meter Run															
702	3 Rounds for time of:															
	- Run 1000-meters															
	- 50 Sit-ups															
703	Complete as many rounds as possible in 8 minutes of:															
	- 10 Back Squats															
	- 10 Strict Chest-to-Bar Pull-Ups															
704	5-4-3-2-1 Reps for time of:															
	- Rope Climbs															
	- Clean and Jerks															
705	5 Rounds for time of:															
	- Run 250-meters															
	- 10 Squats															
	- 10 Push Presses															
706	3 Rounds for time of:															
	- 500-m Row															
	- 25 Thrusters															
	- 15 Pull-Ups															
707	As many reps as possible in 11 minutes:															
	- 11 Overhead Squats															
	- 11 Ball Slams															
	- 11 Wall Ball Shots															
	- 11 Russian Kettlebell Swings															
708	As many reps as possible in 25 minutes:															
	- 10 Pull-Ups															
	- 15 Kettlebell Swings															
	- 20 Box Jumps															
709	Complete as many rounds as possible in 10 minutes of:															
	- 3 Snatches															
	- 6 Clean and Jerks															
	- 9 Ring Rows															
	- 60 Single-unders															
710	For time:															
	- 25 Hang Power Snatches															
	- 25 Push Presses															
	- 25 Sumo Deadlift High Pulls															
	- 25 Front Squats															
711	For time:															
	- 2-minute Elbow Plank															
	- 5 Burpees															
	- 10 Kettlebell Swings															
	- 15 Push-Ups															
	- 20 Goblet Squats															
	- 20 Burpees															
	- 15 Kettlebell Swings															
	- 10 Push-Ups															
	- 5 Goblet Squats															
	- 2-minute Elbow Plank															
	For time:															

		Day 1			Day 2			Day 3			Day 4			Day 5		
	WORKOUTS	Reps	Time	Weight	Reps	Time	Weight	Reps	Time	Weight	Reps	Time	Weight	Reps	Time	Weight
712	- 10 Turkish Get-Ups (Right Arm)															
	- 25 Kettlebell Swings															
	- 10 Overhead Squats (Left Arm)															
	- 25 Kettlebell Swings															
	- 10 Overhead Squats (Right Arm)															
	- 25 Kettlebell Swings															
	- 10 Turkish Get-Ups (Left Arm)															
713	4 Rounds for time:															
	- 25 Kettlebell Swings															
	- 500-meter Run															
714	For time:															
	- 50 Air Squats															
	- 15 Burpees															
	- 40 Sit-Ups															
	- 15 Burpees															
	- 30 Lunges (Alternating Legs)															
	- 15 Burpees															
	- 20 Kettlebell Hang Power Clean (Split between arms)															
	- 15 Burpees															
	- 10 V-ups															
	- 15 Burpees															
	- 20 Kettlebell Swings															
	- 15 Burpees															
	- 30 Lunges (Alternating Legs)															
	- 15 Burpees															
	- 40 Sit-Ups															
	- 15 Burpees															
	- 50 Air Squats															
715	3 Rounds for time of:															
	- 15 Dumbbell Goblet Squats															
	- 20 Burpees															
	- 500-meter Run															
716	2 Rounds for time of:															
	- 20 Dumbbell Walking Lunges															
	- 10 V-ups															
	- 500-meter Run															
717	2 Rounds for time of:															
	30 Dumbbell Squats															
	1 minute plank hold															
	500-meter Run															
718	2 Rounds for time of:															
	20 Dumbbell Romanian Deadlifts															
	20 Push-Ups															
	500-meter Run															
719	For time:															
	- 80 Russian Twists with Dumbbell															
	- 70 Dumbbell Goblet Squats															
	- 60 Dumbbell Push Presses															
	- 50 Dumbbell Reverse Lunges															
	- 40 Dumbbell Snatches (Alternate arms)															
	- 30 Dumbbell Power Cleans															
	- 20 Dumbbell Overhead Squats (Split reps between arms)															
	- 10 Dumbbell Deadlifts															
	For time:															
	- 1000-meter Run															

	WORKOUTS	Day 1			Day 2			Day 3			Day 4			Day 5		
		Reps	Time	Weight	Reps	Time	Weight	Reps	Time	Weight	Reps	Time	Weight	Reps	Time	Weight
720	- 40 Dumbbell Snatches (Alternating arms)															
	- 40 Sit-Ups															
	- 750-meter Run															
	- 30 Dumbbell Snatches (Alternating arms)															
	- 30 Sit-Ups															
	- 500-meter Run															
	- 20 Dumbbell Snatches (Alternating arms)															
	- 20 Sit-Ups															
721	5 Rounds for time of:															
	- 20 Dumbbell Thrusters															
	- 20 Dumbbell Overhead Reverse Lunge (Alternating Legs)															
722	For time:															
	- 20 Dumbbell Thrusters															
	- 500-meter Run															
	- 20 Dumbbell Thrusters															
	- 500-meter Run															
	- 20 Dumbbell Thrusters															
	- 500-meter Run															
723	Every minute on the minute for 20 minutes of:															
	- Odd minutes: 30 Lunges (Alternating Legs and Alternating Front & Reverse Lunges)															
	- Even minutes: 20 Push-Ups															
724	3 Rounds for time of:															
	- 10 Air Squats															
	- 20 Push-Ups															
	- 30 Walking Lunges (Alternating Legs)															
	- 20 Push-Ups															
	- 10 Jumping Jacks															
725	5 Rounds for time:															
	- 10 Sit-ups															
	- 20 Push-Ups															
	- 30 Second Up and down plank															
	- 40 Russian Twists															
	- 50 Mountain Climbers															
	- 60 Jumping Jacks															
	- 70 Air Squats															
726	5 Rounds for time of:															
	- 15 Push-Ups															
	- 30 Sit-ups															
	- 15 Push-Ups															
	- 30 V-ups															
	- 15 Push-Ups															
	- 30 Lunges (Alternating Legs)															
	4 Round for time of:															
	- 20 seconds Burpees															
	10 Second Rest															
	- 20 seconds Russian Twists															
	10 Second Rest															

		Day 1			Day 2			Day 3			Day 4			Day 5		
	WORKOUTS	Reps	Time	Weight	Reps	Time	Weight	Reps	Time	Weight	Reps	Time	Weight	Reps	Time	Weight
	- 20 seconds Lunges (Alternating Legs)															
	10 Second Rest															
727	- 20 seconds Push-Ups															
	10 Second Rest															
	- 20 seconds Mountain Climbers															
	10 Second Rest															
	- 20 seconds Wall Walks															
	10 Second Rest															
	- 20 seconds Air Squats															
	10 Second Rest															
	12 Rounds for time of:															
	- 5 Push-Ups															
728	- 5 Air Squats															
	- 5 Sit-ups															
	5 Rounds for time:															
	- 500-meter Run															
	- 50 Walking Lunges															
729	- 40 Sit-Ups															
	- 30 Push-Ups															
	- 20 Kettlebell Swings															
	- 10 Burpees Over Kettlebell															
	For time:															
	- 300 Kettlebell Swings															
730	*Every minute on the minute: 5 Burpees starting at 01:00															
	20-16-12-8-4 Reps for time:															
	- Kettlebell Cleans (Alternating arms)															
731	- Hand Release Push Ups															
	- Burpees															
	For time:															
	- 200 Russian Kettlebell Swings															
732	- Perform the following every time you put the Kettlebell down:															
	- 15 Air Squats															
	- 10 Push-Ups															
	- 5 Burpees															
	For time:															
	- 1000-meter Run															
	- 20 Kettlebell Snatches															
	- 20 Kettlebell Clean and Push Jerk															
	- 20 Air Squats															
	- 20 Kettlebell Swings															
733	- 20 V-ups															
	- 20 Burpees															
	- 20 Air Squats															
	- 20 Push-Ups															
	- 20 V-ups															
	- 20 Kettlebell Swings															
	3 Rounds for time of:															
	- 10 Dumbbell Snatches (Right arm)															
	- 10 Dumbbell Overhead Lunges (Right arm)															
	- 10 Dumbbell Snatches (Left arm)															

	WORKOUTS	Day 1			Day 2			Day 3			Day 4			Day 5		
		Reps	Time	Weight	Reps	Time	Weight	Reps	Time	Weight	Reps	Time	Weight	Reps	Time	Weight
734	- 10 Dumbbell Overhead Lunges (Left arm)															
	- 10 Dumbbell Power Cleanse															
	- 10 Dumbbell Front Squats															
	- 10 Dumbbell Power Cleans															
	- 10 Dumbbell Front Squats															
735	5 Rounds for time of:															
	- 10 Dumbbell Thrusters															
	- 20 Burpees															
	- 40 Air Squats															
736	3 Rounds for time of:															
	- 1000-meter Run															
	- 30 Burpees															
737	For time:															
	Part 1: Every minute on the minute for 3 minutes of:															
	- 10 Dumbbell Rows (Alternating arms)															
	- 10 Pull-Ups															
	Part 2: Every minute on the minute for 3 minutes of:															
	- 10 Dumbbell Thrusters															
	- 10 Push-Ups															
	Part 3: Every minute on the minute for 3 minutes of:															
	- 10 Dumbbell Rows (Alternating arms)															
	- 10 Air Squats															
	Part 4: As many rounds as possible in 3 minutes of:															
	- Dumbbell Thrusters															
738	21-15-9 Reps for time of:															
	- Dumbbell Thrusters															
	- Burpees															
	- Air Squats															
739	For time:															
	- 300 Air Squats															
740	Every minute on the minute for 21 minutes (each exercise is per minute):															
	- 21 Jump Squats															
	- 21 Push-Ups															
	- 21 Jumping Jacks															
	- 21 V-ups															
	- 21 Burpees															
741	For time:															
	- 100 Jumping Jacks															
	- 90 Front Lunges															
	- 80 Mountain Climbers															
	- 70 Butt Kicks															
	- 60 second Plank															
	- 50 Squats															
	- 40 Bicycle Crunches															
	- 30 Speed skaters															

		Day 1			Day 2			Day 3			Day 4			Day 5		
	WORKOUTS	Reps	Time	Weight	Reps	Time	Weight	Reps	Time	Weight	Reps	Time	Weight	Reps	Time	Weight
	- 20 High Knees															
	- 10 Power Jacks															
	- 5 Burpees															
	Every minute on the minute for 20 minutes:															
742	- 5 Push-Ups															
	- 5 Jump Squats															
	- 5 V-ups															
	- 5 Jumping Jacks															
	5 Rounds for time of:															
	- 30 Squats															
	- 25 Lateral Lunges (Alternating Legs)															
743	- 20 Push-Ups															
	- 15 Fire Hydrants (Alternating Legs)															
	- 10 Mountain Climbers															
	- 5 Burpees															
	As many rounds as possible in 11 minutes of:															
	- 11 Front Lunges (Alternating Legs)															
744	- 11 Lateral Split Squats (Alternating Legs)															
	- 11 Push-Ups															
	- 11 Hip bridges															
	- 11 Mountain Climbers															
	11 Rounds for time of:															
	- 11 Rotational jacks															
	- 11 Crunch Kicks															
745	- 11 Sitting Twists															
	- 11 Raised Leg circles															
	- 11 Butterfly Sit-ups															
	- 11 Wall Walks															
	11-10-9-8-7-6-5-4-3-2-1 Reps for Time:															
	- Sit-Ups															
	- Push-Ups															
	- Air Squats															
746	- Kettlebell Push Press (Split reps between arms)															
	- Kettlebell Snatches (Split reps between arms)															
	- Kettlebell Push Press (Split reps between arms)															
	- Push-Ups															
	For time:															
	- 22 Russian Kettlebell Swings															
	- 22 Single Arm Kettlebell Suitcase Squats (Split reps between arms)															
747	- 22 Sit-Ups															
	- 22 Kettlebell Snatches															
	- 22 Goblet Squats															
	- 22 Push-Ups															
	- 22 American Kettlebell Swings															
	As many rounds as possible in 15 minutes:															
748	- 5 Push-Ups															

		Day 1			Day 2			Day 3			Day 4			Day 5		
	WORKOUTS	Reps	Time	Weight	Reps	Time	Weight	Reps	Time	Weight	Reps	Time	Weight	Reps	Time	Weight
748	- 8 Kettlebell Thruster (Alternating arms)															
	- 11 Kettlebell Deadlifts															
	- 50-meter Kettlebell Goblet Carry															
749	<u>20 Rounds for time:</u>															
	- 6 Burpees															
	- 12 Goblet Squats															
	- 18 Kettlebell Swings															
	- 12 Burpees															
750	<u>For time:</u>															
	- 20 Push-Ups															
	- 10 Kettlebell Swing															
	- 15 Push-Ups															
	- 15 Kettlebell Swing															
	- 10 Push-Ups															
	20 Kettlebell Swing															
	- 5 Push-Ups															
	- 25 Kettlebell Swing															
751	<u>For time:</u>															
	- 20 Kettlebell Cossack Squat (Alternating legs)															
	- 25 Kettlebell Swing															
	- 20 Kettlebell Cossack Squat (Alternating legs)															
	- 25 Kettlebell Swing															
	- 20 Kettlebell Cossack Squat (Alternating legs)															
	-25 Kettlebell Swing															
	- 20 Kettlebell Cossack Squat (Alternating legs)															
	- 25 Kettlebell Swing															
752	<u>3 Rounds for time:</u>															
	- 20 Air Squats															
	- 20 Push-Ups															
	- 20 Kettlebell Squat															
	- 20 One Arm Kettlebell Swings (Split reps between arms)															
753	<u>As many rounds as possible in 20 minutes of:</u>															
	- 20 Air Squats															
	- 20 Dumbbell Rows (Right arm)															
	- 20 Mountain Climbers															
	- 20 Dumbbell Rows (Left arm)															
	- 20 Sit-ups															
754	<u>5 Rounds of:</u>															
	- 10 Burpees															
	- 20 Dumbbell Thrusters															
	- 30 Plank Shoulder Taps															
755	<u>Every minute on the minute for 15 minutes of:</u>															
	- 10 Dumbbell Snatches (Alternating arms)															
	*After each 3 minutes perform															
	- 50 Jumping Jacks															
756	<u>10 Rounds for time of:</u>															
	- 200-meter Run															
	- 15 Dumbbell Burpee Deadlifts															
757	<u>13 Rounds for time of:</u>															
	- 13 Dumbbell Hang Squat Cleans															
	- 13 Push-Ups															
758	<u>5 Rounds for time of:</u>															
	- 10 Dumbbell Man-Makers															
	- 20 Dumbbell Deadlifts															
	- 30 Dumbbell Snatches (Split reps between arms)															

		Day 1			Day 2			Day 3			Day 4			Day 5		
	WORKOUTS	Reps	Time	Weight	Reps	Time	Weight	Reps	Time	Weight	Reps	Time	Weight	Reps	Time	Weight
	- 40 Overhead Lunges (Split reps between arms)															
	- 50 Dumbbell Swings															
	21-15-9 Reps for time of:															
	- Dumbbell Thrusters															
759	- Air Squats															
	- Burpees															
	- Push-Ups															
	For time:															
	- 8 Dumbbell Bent Over Rows															
	- 8 Dumbbell Ground-to-Overheads (Split reps between arms)															
	- 8 Up-Downs + Mountain Climbers															
760	- 8 Dumbbell Bent Over Rows															
	- 8 Dumbbell Ground-to-Overheads															
	- 8 Up-Downs + Mountain Climbers															
	- 8 Dumbbell Bent Over Rows															
	- 8 Dumbbell Ground-to-Overheads															
	- 8 Up-Downs + Mountain Climbers															
	5 Rounds for time of:															
	- 20 Dumbbell Thrusters															
761	- 250-meter Run															
	- 20 Burpees															
	For time:															
762	- 30 Dumbbell Devil Presses															
	- 50 Dumbbell Thrusters															
	- 60 Burpees															
	As many rounds as possible in 25 minutes of:															
	- 5 Dumbbell Thrusters															
763	- 5 Push-Ups															
	- 5 Dumbbell Deadlifts															
	- 5 Pull-Ups															
	- 5 Dumbbell Devil Presses															
	For time:															
764	- 100 Burpees															
	- 100 Push-Ups															
	- 100 Air Squats															
	5 Rounds for time of:															
	- 20 Air Squats															
765	- 20 Lunges (Alternating Legs)															
	- 20 Push-Ups															
	- 20 Squat Jumps															
	Every minute on the minute for 10 minutes:															
766	- 5 Push Ups															
	- 5 Air Squats															
	- 5 Burpees															
	For time:															
	- 11 Jump Squat															
	- 11 Push ups															
	- 11 Jumping Lunges															
	- 11 Bicycle Crunches															
767	- 11 Burpees															
	- 11 Reverse Lunges (Alternating Legs)															
	- 11 Air Squats															
	- 11 Sit-ups															
	- 11 Front Lunges (Alternating Legs)															
	- 11 Box Jumps															
	As many as rounds as possible in 18 minutes of:															

	WORKOUTS	Day 1			Day 2			Day 3			Day 4			Day 5		
		Reps	Time	Weight	Reps	Time	Weight	Reps	Time	Weight	Reps	Time	Weight	Reps	Time	Weight
768	- 6 Squats															
	- 6 Burpees															
	- 6 Side Lunges (Alternating Legs)															
	- 6 Push-Ups															
	- 6 Glute bridges															
769	5 Round for time of:															
	- 11 Push-Ups															
	- 11 Air Squat															
	- 11 Front Lunges (Alternating Legs)															
	- 11 Sit-ups															
	- 11 Burpees															
770	5 Round for time of:															
	- 25 Push-Ups															
	- 25 Air Squats															
	- 25 Walking Lunges															
	- 25 Jumping Jacks															
771	For time:															
	- 100 Burpees															
	- 100 Sit-ups															
	- 100 Push-Ups															
772	5 Round for time of:															
	- 12 Air Squats															
	- 12 Push-Ups															
	- 12 Jumping Jacks															
	- 12 Burpees															
	- 12 Front Lunges (Alternating Legs)															
773	3 Round for time of:															
	- 30 Push-Ups															
	- 30 Crunches															
	- 30 Squats															
774	As many rounds as possible in 25 minutes:															
	- 5 Wall Walks															
	- 10 Push-Ups															
	- 15 Jumping Jacks															
	- 20 Mountain Climbers															
	- 25 Reverse Lunges (Alternating Legs)															
775	3 Rounds for time:															
	- 500-meter Run															
	- 30 American Kettlebell Swings															
	- 20 Kettlebell Single Arm Front Rack Lunge (Split reps between arms)															
	- 10 Burpees Over Kettlebell															
	- 20 Kettlebell Thruster (Split reps between arms)															
	- 30 V-Ups															
	- 500-meter Run															
776	For time:															
	- 50 Air Squats															
	- 10 Burpees															
	- 40 Sit-ups															
	- 10 Burpees															
	- 30 Kettlebell Clean Squat Press (Split reps between arms)															
	- 10 Burpees															
	- 20 Kettlebell Swings															
	- 10 Burpees															
	- 10 meter Bear Crawl															
	- 10 Burpees															
	- 20 Kettlebell Swings															
	- 10 Burpees															
	- 30 Kettlebell Clean Squat Press (Split reps between arms)															
	50-40-30-20-10 Reps for time:															

		Day 1			Day 2			Day 3			Day 4			Day 5		
	WORKOUTS	Reps	Time	Weight	Reps	Time	Weight	Reps	Time	Weight	Reps	Time	Weight	Reps	Time	Weight
777	- Kettlebell Swings															
	- Kettlebell Goblet Squats															
778	Every minute on the minute for 10 minutes of:															
	- 10 Single Arm Kettlebell Swings (Right arm)															
	- 10 Single Arm Kettlebell Swings (Left arm)															
	- 10 Burpees															
779	As many rounds as possible in 10 minutes:															
	- 5 Kettlebell Clean and Press (Per arm)															
	- 5 Kettlebell Clean and Squat (Per arm)															
	- 5 Single-Arm Kettlebell Swings (Per arm)															
	- 5 Kettlebell Snatches (Per arm)															
780	6 Rounds for time:															
	- 20 Kettlebell Swings															
	- 20 Burpees															
781	As many rounds as possible in 10															
	- 5 Burpees															
	- 10 Kettlebell Deadlifts															
	- 20 Goblet Squats															
	- 30 Kettlebell Swings															
782	For time:															
	- 22 Kettlebell Clean Reverse Lunge (Alternating arms)															
	- 20 Kettlebell Push Press (Alternating arms)															
	- 18 Kettlebell Goblet Squat															
	16 Kettlebell V Ups															
	- 14 Kettlebell Deadlift High-pulls															
783	As many rounds as possible in 25 minutes:															
	- 5 Burpees															
	- 15 Push-Ups															
	- 30 Kettlebell Swings															
784	As many rounds as possible in 15 minutes:															
	- 5 Pull-Ups															
	- 10 Push-Ups															
	- 15 Air Squats															
785	For time:															
	- 100 Pull-Ups															
	- 100 Push-Ups															
	- 100 Sit-ups															
	- 100 Squats															
786	For time: 21-15-9 Reps of															
	- Thrusters															
	- Pull-Ups															
	- Air Squats															
787	3 Rounds for time of:															
	- 400-meter Run															
	- 30 Kettlebell Swings															
	- 20 Pull-Ups															
788	4 Rounds for time of:															
	- 400-meter Run															
	- 20 Overhead Squats															
789	21-15-9 Reps for time of:															
	- Deadlifts															
	- Push-Ups															
790	For time:															
	- 40 Clean and Jerks															
791	For time:															

		Day 1			Day 2			Day 3			Day 4			Day 5		
	WORKOUTS	Reps	Time	Weight	Reps	Time	Weight	Reps	Time	Weight	Reps	Time	Weight	Reps	Time	Weight
791	- 40 Snatches															
	For time:															
	- 500-meter Run															
	- 100 Pull-Ups															
792	- 200 Push-Ups															
	- 300 Squats															
	- 500-meter Run															
	5 Rounds for time of:															
793	- 500-meter Run															
	- 20 Overhead Squats															
	For time:															
794	- 1000-meter Row															
	- 60 Thrusters															
	- 40 Pull-Ups															
	For time:															
795																
	- 200 Wall Balls															
	21-15-9 Reps for time of:															
796	- Clean															
	- Squat															
	21-15-9 Reps for time of:															
	- Push-Ups															
797	- Dumbbell Squat Snatches (Alternating arms)															
	- Push-Ups															
	6 Rounds for time of:															
	- 12 Deadlifts															
798	- 9 Hang Power Cleans															
	- 6 Push Jerks															
	5 Rounds for time of:															
799	- 500-meter Run															
	- 25 Kettlebell Swings															
	- 25 Pull-Ups															
	3 Rounds for time of:															
	- 1 minute Wall Balls															
	- 1 minute Sumo Deadlift high-pull															
800	- 1 minute Box Jumps															
	- 1 minute Calorie Row															
	- 1 minute Push press															
	- 1 minute Rest															
	For time:															
801	- 50 Power Snatches															
	11-9-7 Reps for time of:															
802	- Front Squats															
	- Squat Snatches															
	For time:															
803	- 200 Kettlebell Swings															
	3 Rounds for time of:															
804	- 500-meter Run															

		Day 1			Day 2			Day 3			Day 4			Day 5		
	WORKOUTS	Reps	Time	Weight	Reps	Time	Weight	Reps	Time	Weight	Reps	Time	Weight	Reps	Time	Weight
804	- 30 Kettlebell Swings - 12 Kettlebell Goblet Squats															
805	For time: - 11 Kettlebell Snatches (each arm), then 10 reps (each arm), down to 1 rep (each arm)															
806	For time: - 11 Kettlebell Clean and Jerk (each arm), then 10 reps (each arm), down to 1 rep (each arm)															
807	For time: - 10 Kettlebell Thrusters each arm, then 9 reps each arm, down to 1 rep each arm															
808	For time: - 10 Kettlebell Goblet Squats, then 9 reps, down to 1 rep															
809	6 Rounds for time of: - 12 Kettlebell Man Makers															
810	5 Rounds for time of: - 10 Kettlebell Deadlifts															
811	For time: - 120m Farmers Carry with two Kettlebells															
812	3 Rounds for time of: - 6 Kettlebell Turkish Get-ups (Per each arm)															
813	21-15-9 Reps for time of: - Thruster - Push-Ups															
814	For time 9 Reps of each exercise, then 8 reps, down to 1 rep: - Deadlifts - Hang Power Cleans - Push Presses - Front Squats															
815	For time: - 30 Deadlifts - 30 Snatch															
816	For time: - 35 Clean and Jerks															
817	21-15-9 Reps for time of: - Deadlifts - Push-Ups															
818	5 Rounds for time of: - 500-meter Run - 30 Plate Ground to Overhead - 10 Handstand Push-Ups															
819	40-30-20-10 Reps for time of: - Double unders - Squats - Sit-ups															
820	As many rounds as possible in 9 minutes of: - 3 Power Cleans - 6 Push-Ups															

	WORKOUTS	Day 1			Day 2			Day 3			Day 4			Day 5		
		Reps	Time	Weight	Reps	Time	Weight	Reps	Time	Weight	Reps	Time	Weight	Reps	Time	Weight
	- 9 Air Squats															
821	As many rounds as possible in 20 minute of:															
	- 2 Push-Ups															
	- 4 Push-Ups															
	- 8 Kettlebell Swings															
822	5 Rounds for time of:															
	- 150m Plate Push															
823	8 Rounds for time of:															
	- 8 Handstand Push-Ups															
	- 8 Thrusters															
	- 8 Knees-to-elbows															
824	9 Rounds for time of:															
	- 9 Deadlifts															
	- 9 Burpees															
	- 9 Kettlebell Swings															
	- 9 Pull-Ups															
825	5 Rounds for time of:															
	- 20 Plate Sit Ups to Press															
826	5 Rounds for time of:															
	- 20 Plate Overhead Lunges															
827	3 Rounds for time of:															
	- 20 Hand Power Cleans															
	- 20 Deadlifts															
	- 20 Push Jerk															
828	5 Rounds for time of:															
	- 20 Plate Squats															
	- 20 Plate Push Press															
829	5 Rounds for time of:															
	- 20 Box Jumps															
830	6 Rounds for time of:															
	- 20 Plate bent-Over Rows															
831	For time:															
	- 60 Russian Kettlebell Swings															
	- 30 Goblet Squats															
	- 60 American Kettlebell Swings															
832	4 Rounds for time of:															
	- 400-meter Run															
	- 40 Plate Ground to Overhead															
833	For time: 21-15-9 Reps of															
	- Deadlifts															
	- Power Cleans															
834	For time: 21-15-9 Reps of															
	- Push-Ups															
	- Clean and jerks															
	- Burpees															
	For time:															

		Day 1			Day 2			Day 3			Day 4			Day 5		
	WORKOUTS	Reps	Time	Weight	Reps	Time	Weight	Reps	Time	Weight	Reps	Time	Weight	Reps	Time	Weight
835	- 1000m Run - 30 Kettlebell Swings - 30 Pull-Ups															
836	For time: - 30 Dumbbell Lunges (Alternate legs) - 50 Sit-Ups															
837	4 Rounds for time of: - 20 Burpees - 20 Hand Release Push-Ups - 20 Dumbbell Deadlifts															
838	For time: 21-15-9 Reps of - Hand Release Push-Ups - Burpees															
839	5 Rounds for time of: - 40 Sit-Ups - 40 Dumbbell Lunges (Alternate legs)															
840	4 Rounds for time of: - 500-meter Run - 20 Back Squats															
841	5 Rounds for time: - 20 Walkout Push-Ups - 20 Squat Jumps															
842	For time: - 40 Goblet Squats - 40 V-ups - 40 Kettlebell Bent Over Row (Alternating arms)															
843	For time: - 20 Push-Ups - 20 V-ups - 20 Air Squats															
844	10 Rounds for time of: - 500-meter Run Rest 1 minute between rounds															
845	5 Rounds for time of: - 20 Walking Lunges - 10 Burpees															
846	6 Rounds for time of: - 500-meter Run - 30 Box Jumps															
847	As many reps as possible in 20 minutes: - 10 Deadlifts - 20 Box Jumps - 30 Push-Ups															
848	For time: - 30 Lunges (Alternating legs) - 20 Burpees															
849	4 Rounds for time of: - 25 Kettlebell Swings - 25 Burpees - 25 meter Bear Crawl															
850	For time: - 15 Snatch Push Press + Overhead Squat - 20 Kettlebell Swings - 25 Burpees															
851	For time: - 35 Lunges (Alternating legs) - 25 Hand Clean - 15 Burpees															
852	For time: - 50 Sit-Ups - 25 Burpees															

		Day 1			Day 2			Day 3			Day 4			Day 5		
	WORKOUTS	Reps	Time	Weight	Reps	Time	Weight	Reps	Time	Weight	Reps	Time	Weight	Reps	Time	Weight
	- 50 Air Squats															
853	9-12-15 Reps for time of:															
	- Burpees															
	- Kettlebell Swings															
854	For time:															
	- 100 Kettlebell Swings															
	- 100 Air Squats															
855	For time:															
	- 100 Sit-Ups															
	- 100 Push-Ups															
856	40-20-10 Reps for time of:															
	- Air Squats															
	- Burpees															
857	5 Rounds for time of:															
	- 10 Sit-ups															
	- 20 Deadlift															
	- 30 Burpees															
	- 40 Jumping Jacks															
858	As many reps as possible in 25 minutes:															
	- 60 Jumping Ropes															
	- 20 Power Snatches															
859	Every minute on the minute for 10 minutes:															
	- 10 Burpees															
	- 10 Thrusters															
860	As many rounds as possible in 22 minutes:															
	- 16 Kettlebell Deadlifts															
	- 19 Air Squats															
861	Every minute on the minute for 20															
	- Odd minutes - 20 Burpees															
	- Even minutes - 30 Kettlebell Swings															
862	For time:															
	- 500-meter Run															
	- 50 Push-Ups															
	- 500-meter Run															
863	For time:															
	- 40 Goblet Squats															
	- 500-meter Run															
	- 40 Push-Ups															
864	As many rounds as possible in 25 minutes:															
	- 20 Push-Ups															
	- 25 Kettlebell Swings															
	- 30 Mountain Climbers															
865	11 Rounds for time:															
	- 11 Air Squats															
	- 11 Kettlebell Deadlifts															
866	For time:															
	- 21 Thrusters															
	- 9 Deadlifts															
	- 15 Thrusters															
	- 15 Deadlifts															
	- 9 Thrusters															
	- 21 Deadlifts															

		Day 1			Day 2			Day 3			Day 4			Day 5		
	WORKOUTS	Reps	Time	Weight	Reps	Time	Weight	Reps	Time	Weight	Reps	Time	Weight	Reps	Time	Weight
867	<u>5 Rounds for time:</u>															
	- 30 Single-Arm Kettlebell Swings (Split reps between arms)															
	- 30 Air Squats															
	- 30 Burpees															
868	<u>4 Rounds for time:</u>															
	- 30 Single-Arm Kettlebell Overhead Squats (Split reps between arms)															
	- 30 Push-Ups															
869	<u>For time:</u>															
	- 40 Dumbbell Power Snatches (Split reps between arms)															
	- 20-meter Dumbbell Overhead Walking Lunges (Per arm)															
	- 40 Dumbbell Overhead Squats (Alternate arms every 10 reps)															
	- 20-meter Dumbbell Overhead Walking Lunges (Per arm)															
870	<u>For time:</u>															
	- 20 Dumbbell Hang Clean-and-Jerks															
	- 20-meter Dumbbell Overhead Walking Lunges (Per arm)															
	- 20 Dumbbell Squat Cleans															
	- 20-meter Dumbbell Overhead Walking Lunges (Per arm)															
	- 20 Dumbbell Squat Snatches (Split reps between arms)															
871	<u>5 Rounds for time of:</u>															
	- 50 Sit-ups															
	- 50 Jumping Jacks															
872	<u>5 Rounds for time:</u>															
	- 30 Air Squats															
	- 60 Jumping Jacks															
873	<u>As many rounds as possible in 12 minutes of:</u>															
	- 10 Hand Power Cleans															
	- 10 Push-Ups															
874	<u>4 Rounds for time of:</u>															
	- 20 Reverse Lunges (Alternating legs)															
	- 40 Push-Ups															
	- 60 Air Squats															
875	<u>3 rounds of 1 minute each of:</u>															
	- Thrusters															
	- Power Snatches															
	- Overhead Squats															
	- Rowing															
876	<u>5 Rounds for time of:</u>															
	- 20 Kettlebell Swings															
	- 20 Box Jumps															
	- 500-meter Run															
	- 20 Burpees															
	- 20 Wall Ball Shots															
	<u>For time:</u>															
	- 100-meter Run															

	WORKOUTS	Day 1			Day 2			Day 3			Day 4			Day 5		
		Reps	Time	Weight	Reps	Time	Weight	Reps	Time	Weight	Reps	Time	Weight	Reps	Time	Weight
877	- 15 Thrusters - 25 Burpees - 50 Box Step-Ups															
878	For time: - 30 Pull-Ups - 50 Thrusters - 1000m Row															
879	For time: - 150 Wall Balls															
880	5 rounds of max reps of: - Bench press - Pull-Ups - Squats															
881	As many rouds as possible in 24 minutes of : - 2 Muscle-ups - 4 Handstand Push-Ups - 8 Kettlebell Swings - 16 Double unders															
882	5 Rounds of 5 reps each of: - Hang Power Cleans - Deadlifts - Front Squats - Push presses - Back Squats without putting the Barbell down within a round															
883	As many rounds as possible in 15 minutes: - 9 Burpees -12 Push-Ups - 15 Mountain Climbers															
884	As many rounds as possible in 12 minutes: - 3 Air Squats - 9 Pull-Ups - 12 Power Jacks															
885	For time: - 50 Air Squats - 50 Pull-Ups - 50 Push-Ups															
886	For time: - 25 Push-Ups - 50 Air Squats - 25 Push-Ups - 50 Air Squats															
887	6 Rounds for time: - 6 Kettlebell Squats - 6 V-ups - 6 Kettlebell Lunges															

	WORKOUTS	Day 1			Day 2			Day 3			Day 4			Day 5		
		Reps	Time	Weight	Reps	Time	Weight	Reps	Time	Weight	Reps	Time	Weight	Reps	Time	Weight
888	For time: - 500-meter Run - 50 Russian Kettlebell Swings - 50 Kettlebell Taters - 250-meter Run - 25 Russian Kettlebell Swings															
889	For time: - 30 Kettlebell Taters - 200-meter Run - 20 Russian Kettlebell Swings - 20 Kettlebell Taters															
890	For time: - 100-meter Run - 25 Russian Kettlebell Swings - 25 Kettlebell Taters															
891	4 Rounds of 1 minute each of max effort: - Thrusters - Front Squats - Deadlifts 1 minute Rest between rounds															
892	For time of: - 100 Curtis P's 1 "Curtis P" complex is comprised of 1 Power Clean, 1 Lunge (each leg), & 1 Push Press															
893	For time: 25 reps of: - Front Squats - Deadlifts - Hang Power Cleans - Push presses - Back Squats															
894	For time: - 5 Pull-ups - 500 meter Run - 20 Thrusters - 800 meter Run - 20 Thrusters - 500 meter Run - 50 Pull-Ups															
895	Every minute on the minute for 20 minutes: - 5 Deadlifts - 5 Hang Power Cleans - 5 Front Squats															
896	3 Rounds for time of: - 3 Deadlifts - 3 Hang Power Cleans - 3 Front Squats - 3 Push presses - 3 Back Squats 1 minute rest between rounds															
897	9-87-6-5-4-3-2-1 Reps of: - Deadlifts - Hang Power Cleans - Front Squats - Push presses - Back Squats															
898	As many rounds as possible in 10 minutes of: - 3 Deadlifts - 3 Hang Power Cleans - 3 Front Squats															
899	For time: - 500-meter Run															

		Day 1			Day 2			Day 3			Day 4			Day 5		
	WORKOUTS	Reps	Time	Weight	Reps	Time	Weight	Reps	Time	Weight	Reps	Time	Weight	Reps	Time	Weight
	- 50 Kettlebell Swings															
	As many rounds as possible in 20 minutes of:															
	- 20 Air Squats															
900	- 20 Kettlebell Push Press (Alternating															
	- 200-meter Run															
	- 20 Kettlebell Swings															
	For time:															
	- 25 Burpees															
901	- 25 Air Squats															
	- 25 Single-Arm Kettlebell Push Press															
	- 500-meter Run															
	As many rounds as possible in 18 minutes of:															
902	- 3 Burpees															
	- 6 Air Squats															
	- 9 Push-Ups															
	5 Rounds for time of:															
903	- 15 Kettlebell Deadlifts															
	- 50-meter Kettlebell Farmer's Carry															
	4 Rounds for time of:															
904	- 15 Kettlebell Thrusters															
	- 20 meter Kettlebell Farmer's Carry															
	As many rounds as possible in 15 minutes:															
905	- 25 Speed skaters															
	- 25 Plank Jacks															
	5 Rounds for time of:															
906	- 20 Russian Twists															
	- 20 Reverse Crunches															
	As many rounds as possible in 20 minutes:															
907	- 20 Air Squats															
	- 20 High Knees															
	5 rounds for time of:															
908	- 500-m run															
	- 30 Kettlebell Snatches (Split reps between arms)															
	5 Rounds for time of:															
909	- 30 Jumping Jacks															
	- 20 Tricep Dips															
	- 10 Squats															
	4 Round for time of:															
	- 50 Mountain Climbers															
910	- 20 V-Ups															
	- 20 Push-Ups															
	As many rounds as possible in 15 minutes of:															
911	- 5 Sit-Ups															
	- 5 Hand Release Push-Ups															
	5 Round for time of:															
	- 50 Mountain Climbers															
912																

	WORKOUTS	Day 1			Day 2			Day 3			Day 4			Day 5		
		Reps	Time	Weight	Reps	Time	Weight	Reps	Time	Weight	Reps	Time	Weight	Reps	Time	Weight
912	- 20 V-Ups															
	- 20 Push-Ups															
913	5 Rounds for time of:															
	- 6 Push Jerks															
	- 9 Hang Power Cleans															
	- 12 Deadlifts															
914	As many rounds as possible in 24 minutes of:															
	- 4 Dumbbell Thrusters															
	- 6 Toes-to-Bar															
	- 24 Double-Unders															
915	3 Round for time of:															
	- 60 Jumping Jacks															
	- 30 Cross body punches															
	- 30 Donkey Kicks (Alternating legs)															
916	For time:															
	- 60 Air Squats															
	- 60 Russian Twists															
	- 60 Bicycle Crunches															
	- 60-second Plank															
917	As many rounds as possible in 15 minutes of:															
	- 60 Jumping ropes															
	- 15 Power Snatches															
918	5 Rounds for time of:															
	- 500-meter Run															
	- 15 Overhead Squats															
919	4 Rounds for time of:															
	- 100 Jumping Jacks															
	- 20 Push-Ups															
	- 60-second High Knees (Alternating legs)															
920	21-18-15-12-9-6-3 Reps for time of:															
	- Burpees															
	- Thrusters															
921	As many rounds as possible in 12 minutes of :															
	- 4 Burpees															
	- 4 Push-Ups															
922	As many rounds as possible in 10 minutes of:															
	- 3 Burpees															
	- 10 Power Snatches															
923	9 Rounds for time of:															
	- 3 Squats															
	- 6 Power Jacks															
	- 9 Push-Ups															

		Day 1			Day 2			Day 3			Day 4			Day 5		
	WORKOUTS	Reps	Time	Weight	Reps	Time	Weight	Reps	Time	Weight	Reps	Time	Weight	Reps	Time	Weight
924	For time:															
	- 60-second Up and down plank															
	- 60 Air Squats															
	- 50 Sit-ups															
	- 40 Glute Bridges															
	- 30 Supermans															
925	10 Rounds for time of:															
	- 10 Air Squats															
	- 3 Power Snatches															
926	For time:															
	- 20 Dumbbell Hang Clean															
	- 20 Dumbbell Squats															
	- 20 Dumbbell Push Jerk															
	- 20 Dumbbell Bent Over Rows															
	- 20 Dumbbell Hang Clean															
	- 20 Dumbbell Squats															
	- 20 Dumbbell Push Jerk															
	- 20 Bent Over Rows															
927	As many rounds as possible in 16 minutes of:															
	- 4 Burpees															
	- 4 Dumbbell Thruster															
	- 4 Dumbbell Deadlift															
	- 8 Dumbbell Power Snatch (Split reps between arms)															
928	For time:															
	- 30 Dumbbell Swings															
	- 30 Dumbbell Snatch To Reverse Lunge (Split reps between arms)															
	- 30 Dumbbell Devils Press (Split reps between arms)															
	- 1000-meter Run															
929	For Time:															
	- 15 Overhead Squats															
	- 15 Chest-to-Bar Pull-Ups															
	- 15 Sumo Deadlift High Pulls															
930	For time:															
	- 100 Dumbbell Devil Presses															
931	For time:															
	- 30 Air Squats															
	- 30 Dumbbell Devil Presses															
	- 30 Air Squats															
932	5 Rounds for time of:															
	- 6 Dumbbell Devil Presses															
	- 30 Air Squats															
933	For Time:															
	- 20-Calorie Row															
	- 20 Handstand Push-Ups															

		Day 1			Day 2			Day 3			Day 4			Day 5		
	WORKOUTS	Reps	Time	Weight	Reps	Time	Weight	Reps	Time	Weight	Reps	Time	Weight	Reps	Time	Weight
	- 20 Back Squats															
	- 20 Chest-to-Bar Pull-Ups															
934	For time:															
	- 60 Dumbbell Snatches (Split reps between arms)															
	- 60 Air Squats															
	- 30 Dumbbell Snatches (Split reps between arms)															
	- 30 Air Squats															
935	For time:															
	- 25 Air Squats															
	- 25 Dumbbell Snatches (Alternating arms)															
	- 20 Air Squats															
	- 20 Dumbbell Snatches (Alternating arms)															
	- 15 Air Squats															
	- 15 Dumbbell Snatches (Alternating arms)															
936	5 Rounds for time:															
	- 3 minute Max Push-Ups															
	- 3 minute Max Dumbbell Renegade Rows															
	- 3 minute Max Mountain Climbers															
937	For time:															
	- 30 Turkish Get-ups (Alternating arms)															
938	For time:															
	- 50 Alternating Dumbbell Snatches															
	- 50 Burpee Box Jump Overs															
	- 50 Alternating Dumbbell Snatches															
939	For time:															
	- 500-meter Run															
	- 40 Air Squats															
	- 30 Sit-Ups															
	- 20 Push-Ups															
	- 10 Burpees															
	- 5 V-Ups															
940	For time:															
	- 1000-meter Run															
	- 50 Box Jumps															
	- 50 Wall Ball Shots															
941	For time:															
	- 15 Dumbbell Snatches (Split reps between arms)															
	- 20 Burpees															
	- 25 Dumbbell Snatches (Split reps between arms)															
	- 30 Burpees															
942	21-15-9 Reps for time of:															
	- Dumbbell Snatches (Split reps between arms)															
	- Burpees															
943	Every minute on the minute for 20 minutes:															
	- 1 Power Snatches															

		Day 1			Day 2			Day 3			Day 4			Day 5		
	WORKOUTS	Reps	Time	Weight	Reps	Time	Weight	Reps	Time	Weight	Reps	Time	Weight	Reps	Time	Weight
	- 1 Power Cleans															
944	For time: - 3 Hang Cleans - 3 Front Squats - 3 Shoulder-to-Overheads - 2 Hang Cleans - 2 Front Squats - 2 Shoulder-to-Overheads - 1 Hang Clean - 1 Front Squat - 1 Shoulder-to-Overhead															
945	4 Rounds for time: - 6 Rope Climbs - 12 Toes-to-Bars - 24 Overhead Walking Lunges - 500-meter Run															
946	As many rounds as possible in 20 minutes: - 15 Air Squats - 10 Push-Ups - 5 Burpees															
947	4 Rounds for time of: - 500 meter Row - 10 Power Clean - 15 Toes-to-bar															
948	For time: - 30 Russian Kettlebell Swings - 30 Kettlebell Snatches (Alternating arms) - 30 Kettlebell Cleans (Alternating arms) - 30 American Kettlebell Swings															
949	For time: - 1000-m Run - 50 Kettlebell Swings - 1000-m Run - 50 Kettlebell Swings															
950	For time: - 100 Dumbbell Snatches (Split reps between arms)															
951	As many rounds as possible in 20 minutes: - 500-meter Row - 10 Toes-to-Bars - 15 Burpees															
952	For time: - 30 Dumbbell Snatches - 3 Rope Climbs - 20 Dumbbell Snatches															
	For time:															

		Day 1			Day 2			Day 3			Day 4			Day 5		
	WORKOUTS	Reps	Time	Weight	Reps	Time	Weight	Reps	Time	Weight	Reps	Time	Weight	Reps	Time	Weight
953	- Run 3000 meters (or 15 minutes)															
954	Every minutes on the minutes until you are not able to complete reps															
	- 5 Air Squats															
	- 5 Push-Ups															
	Add 1 rep each round															
955	Every minutes on the minutes for 20 minutes:															
	- 5 Thrusters															
	- 5 Burpees															
	- 5 Toes-to-Bars															
	- 5 Power Snatches															
956	Every minutes on the minutes for 20 minutes:															
	- Odd: 3 Front Squats															
	- Even: 6 Pull-Ups															
957	5 Rounds for time of:															
	- 7 Deadlifts															
	- 6 Burpees															
	- 5 Cleans															
	- 4 Pull-Ups															
	- 3 Thrusters															
	- 2 V-Ups															
958	For Time:															
	- 500-meter Run															
	- 20 Lateral Burpees															
	- 20 Lunges															
	- 20 American Kettlebell Swings															
	- 500-meter Run															
959	For Time:															
	- 60 Burpees															
	- 50 Goblet Squats															
	- 40 Push-Ups															
960	For Time:															
	- 20 Plate Ground to Overhead															
	- 20 Wall Walks															
	- 20 Plate Ground to Overhead															
961	For Time:															
	- 50 Goblet Squats															
	- 50 Burpees															
962	11-9-7-5-3-1 Reps For Time:															
	- Pull-Ups															
	- Squat Cleans															
963	For Time:															
	- 30 Power Clean + Hang Power Clean + Squats															
964	As many rounds as possible in 15 minutes of:															
	- 5 Hang Squat Cleans															
	- 5 Bar-Facing Burpees															
965	As many rounds as possible in 25 minutes of:															
	- 5 Deadlifts															
	- 5 Knees-to-Elbows															
	- 5 Burpees															
	3 Rounds for Time:															

		Day 1			Day 2			Day 3			Day 4			Day 5		
	WORKOUTS	Reps	Time	Weight	Reps	Time	Weight	Reps	Time	Weight	Reps	Time	Weight	Reps	Time	Weight
966	- 1000-meter Run															
	- 30 Chest-to-Bar Pull-Ups															
967	As many rounds as possible in 10 minutes of:															
	- 5 Shoulder-to-Overheads															
	- 5 Deadlifts															
	- 5 Box Jumps															
968	4 Rounds for Time															
	- 30/20-Calorie Row															
	- 25 Ring Push-Ups															
	- 20 Deadlifts															
	- 15 Burpees to Plate															
969	For Time:															
	- 500-meter Run															
	- 80 Front Squats															
	- 80 Toes-to-Bars															
	- 8 Rope Climbs															
	- 500-meter Run															
970	12-9-6-3 Reps For Time:															
	- Squat Cleans															
	- Pull-Ups															
971	As many rounds as possible in 21 minutes:															
	- 2 Air Squats															
	- 4 Thrusters															
	- 8 Bent Over Rows															
	- 16 Push-Ups															
972	21-18-15-12-9-6-3 Reps of:															
	- Push-Ups															
	- Pull-Ups															
973	20 Rounds for time of:															
	- 4 Pull-Ups															
	- 4 Wall Ball Shots															
	- 4 Pull-Ups															
974	For Time:															
	- 1000-meter Run															
	- 100 Box Step-Ups															
	- 100 Ball Slams															
975	For Time:															
	- 50 Push-Ups															
	- 25 Burpees															
	- 50 Push-Ups															
	- 25 Burpees															
976	As many rounds as possible in 20 minutes:															
	- 10 Pull-Ups															
	- 20 Push-Ups															
	- 30 Air Squats															
977	5 Rounds for time of:															
	- 25 Kettlebell Swings															
	- 15 Wall Balls															

		Day 1			Day 2			Day 3			Day 4			Day 5		
	WORKOUTS	Reps	Time	Weight	Reps	Time	Weight	Reps	Time	Weight	Reps	Time	Weight	Reps	Time	Weight
	- 10 Burpees															
	For Time:															
	- 10-9-8-7-6-5-4-3-2-1 reps of:															
978	- Burpees															
	- V-Ups															
	- Push-Ups															
	As many rounds as possible in 20 minutes:															
979	- 5 Pull-Ups															
	- 10 Push-Ups															
	- 15 Air Squats															
	5 Rounds For Time:															
	- 15 Deadlifts															
980	- 10 Hang Power Cleans															
	- 5 Push Jerks															
	For Time:															
	- 22 Push Presses															
981	- 22 Air Squats															
	- 22 Deadlifts															
	For Time:															
	- 13 Box Jumps															
	- 13 Front Squats															
982	- 13 Calorie Row															
	- 13 Power Snatch															
	- 13 Toes-to-Bars															
	- 13 Back Squats															
	For Time:															
	- 20 Push-Ups															
	- 20-Calorie Assault Bike															
983	- 20 Burpees															
	- 20 Sit-Ups															
	- 20 Wall Ball Shots															
	- 20 V-Ups															
	2 Rounds for time of:															
	- 15 Clean-and-Jerks															
	- 15 Pull-Ups															
984	- 15 Overhead Squats															
	- 15 Kettlebell Swings															
	- 15 Hand Release Push-Ups															
	- 15 Thrusters															
	5 Rounds for Time:															
	- 5 Push-Ups															
	- 5 GHD Sit-Ups															
	- 5 Air Squats															
985	- 5 Pull-Ups															
	- 5 Deadlifts															
	- 5 Hang Power Cleans															
	- 5 Shoulder-to-Overheads															
	- 5 Calorie Row															
	2 Rounds for Time:															
	- 250-meter Run															
986	- 15 Kettlebell Swings															
	- 15 Front Squats															
	- 15 Pull-Ups															
	For Time:															
	- 500-meter Run															
987	- 30 Kettlebell Swings															
	- 30 Pull-Ups															
	- 30 Front Squats															
	For Time:															
	- 1000-meter Run															

		Day 1			Day 2			Day 3			Day 4			Day 5		
	WORKOUTS	Reps	Time	Weight	Reps	Time	Weight	Reps	Time	Weight	Reps	Time	Weight	Reps	Time	Weight
988	- 36 Kettlebell Swings - 36 Pull-Ups - 36 Front Squats															
989	For time: 5 Rounds of: - 25 Dumbbell Thrusters - 200-meter Run															
990	For time : - 100 Push-Ups - 100 Kettlebell Swings - 100 Toes-to-Bars															
991	5 Rounds for Time: - 40 Kettlebell Swings - 35 Push-Ups - 30 Pull-Ups - 25 Box Jumps - 500-meter Run															
992	3 Rounds for Time: - 20 Thrusters - 20 Chest-to-Bar Pull-Ups															
993	For time : - 1000-meter Row - 1000-meter Assault Air Bike - 200 Single-Unders															
994	4 Rounds for time of: - 500-meter Row - 10 Hand Power Clean - 10 Clean and Jerk															
995	For time: 9-12-15-21 Reps of - Box jumps - Push-Ups - Burpees															
996	As many rounds as possible in 20 minutes of: - 1000-meter Row - 10 Toes-to-Bars - 15 Burpees															
997	4 Rounds for Time - 12 Calorie Bike - 15 Thrusters - 18 Kettlebell Swings															
998	For time : - 13 Calorie Bike - 16 Box Jumps - 19 Air Squats - 13 Calorie Bike - 16 Wall Ball Shots - 19 Burpees															
999	For Time : - 200-meter Run - 20 Snatches - 20 Pull-Ups - 20 Medicine Ball Cleans - 20 Elbow Plank to Push-Ups															
1000	As many rounds as possible in 33 minutes of: - 11 Wall Ball Shots - 11 Deadlifts - 11 Air Squats - 11 Overhead Walking Lunges - 11 Box Jumps - 11 Power Cleans															

BONUS No 1 - *LOGGING SHEETS* FOR ALL 1000 WORKOUTS

BONUS No 2 - VIDEOS for ALL EXERCISES

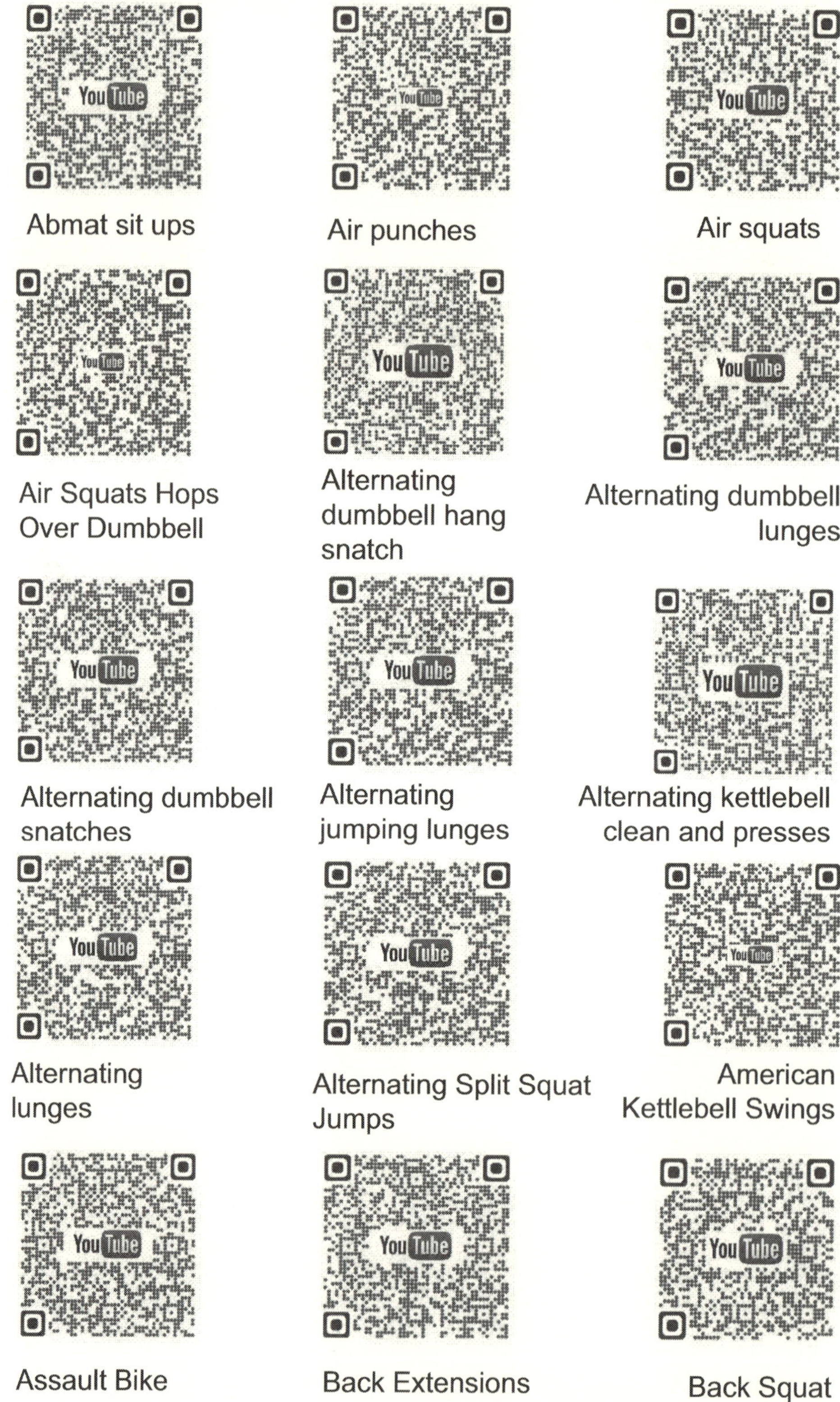

Abmat sit ups

Air punches

Air squats

Air Squats Hops Over Dumbbell

Alternating dumbbell hang snatch

Alternating dumbbell lunges

Alternating dumbbell snatches

Alternating jumping lunges

Alternating kettlebell clean and presses

Alternating lunges

Alternating Split Squat Jumps

American Kettlebell Swings

Assault Bike

Back Extensions

Back Squat

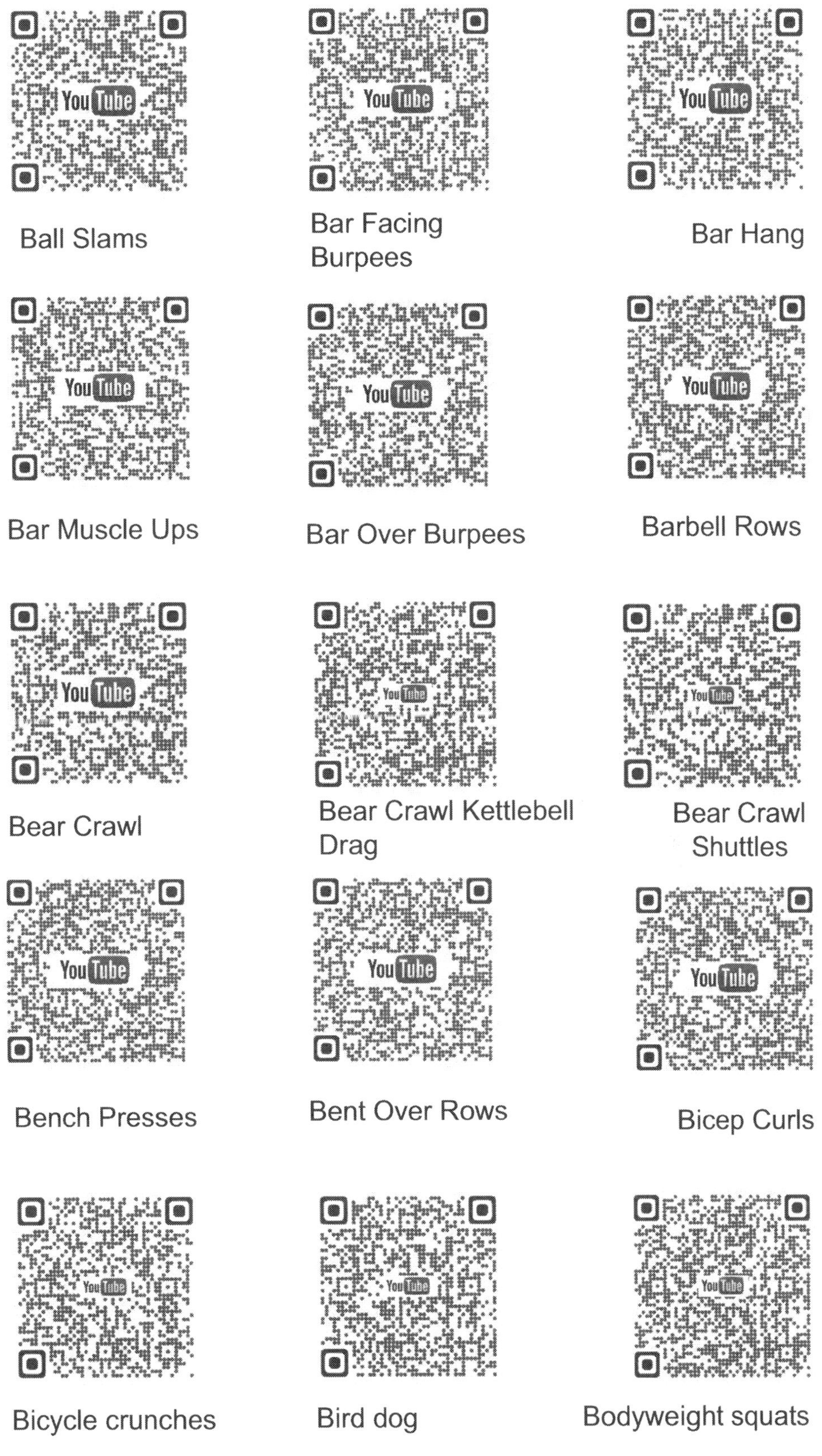

Ball Slams

Bar Facing Burpees

Bar Hang

Bar Muscle Ups

Bar Over Burpees

Barbell Rows

Bear Crawl

Bear Crawl Kettlebell Drag

Bear Crawl Shuttles

Bench Presses

Bent Over Rows

Bicep Curls

Bicycle crunches

Bird dog

Bodyweight squats

Box Jump

Box Jump Overs

Box Step Ups

Bridge

Broad Jump

Burpees

Burpee Box Jump Overs

Burpee Box Jumps

Burpee Box Step Over

Burpee Muscle Ups

Burpees Over Dumbbells

Burpees Over The Bar

Burpee Pull Ups

Butt Kicks

Butterfly sit-ups

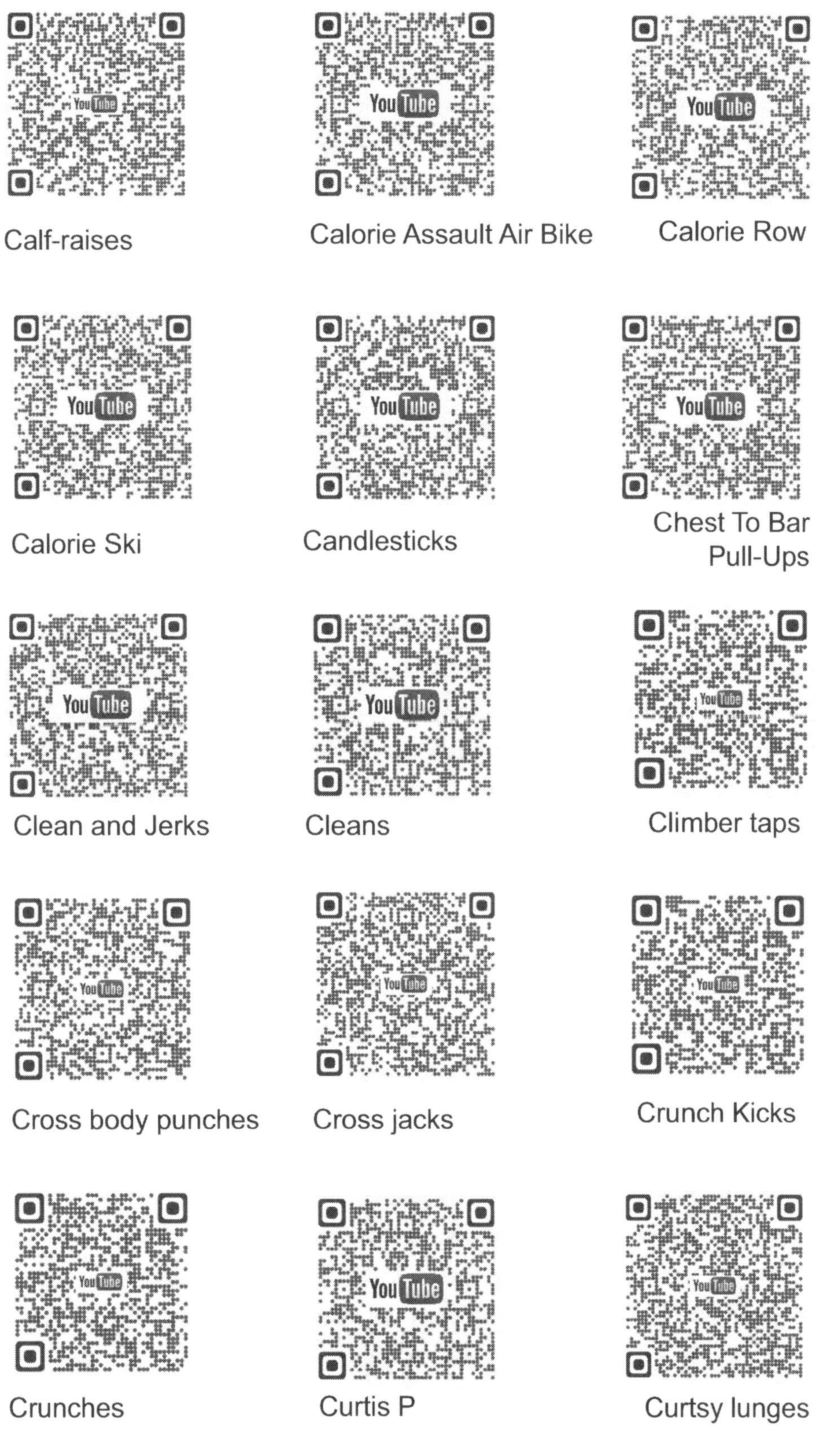
Calf-raises
Calorie Assault Air Bike
Calorie Row
Calorie Ski
Candlesticks
Chest To Bar Pull-Ups
Clean and Jerks
Cleans
Climber taps
Cross body punches
Cross jacks
Crunch Kicks
Crunches
Curtis P
Curtsy lunges

Cossack Squats
Deadlift
Deadlift Burpee Dumbbells
Deficit Handstand Push-Ups
Devil Press Thrusters
Devil Presses
Diamond Push-Ups
Donkey kicks
Double Dumbbell Front Rack Reverse Lunges
Double Kettlebell Swings
Double Under
Down ups
Downward Dog Foot Taps
Downward dog to plank
Dual Dumbbell Overhead Reverse Lunge

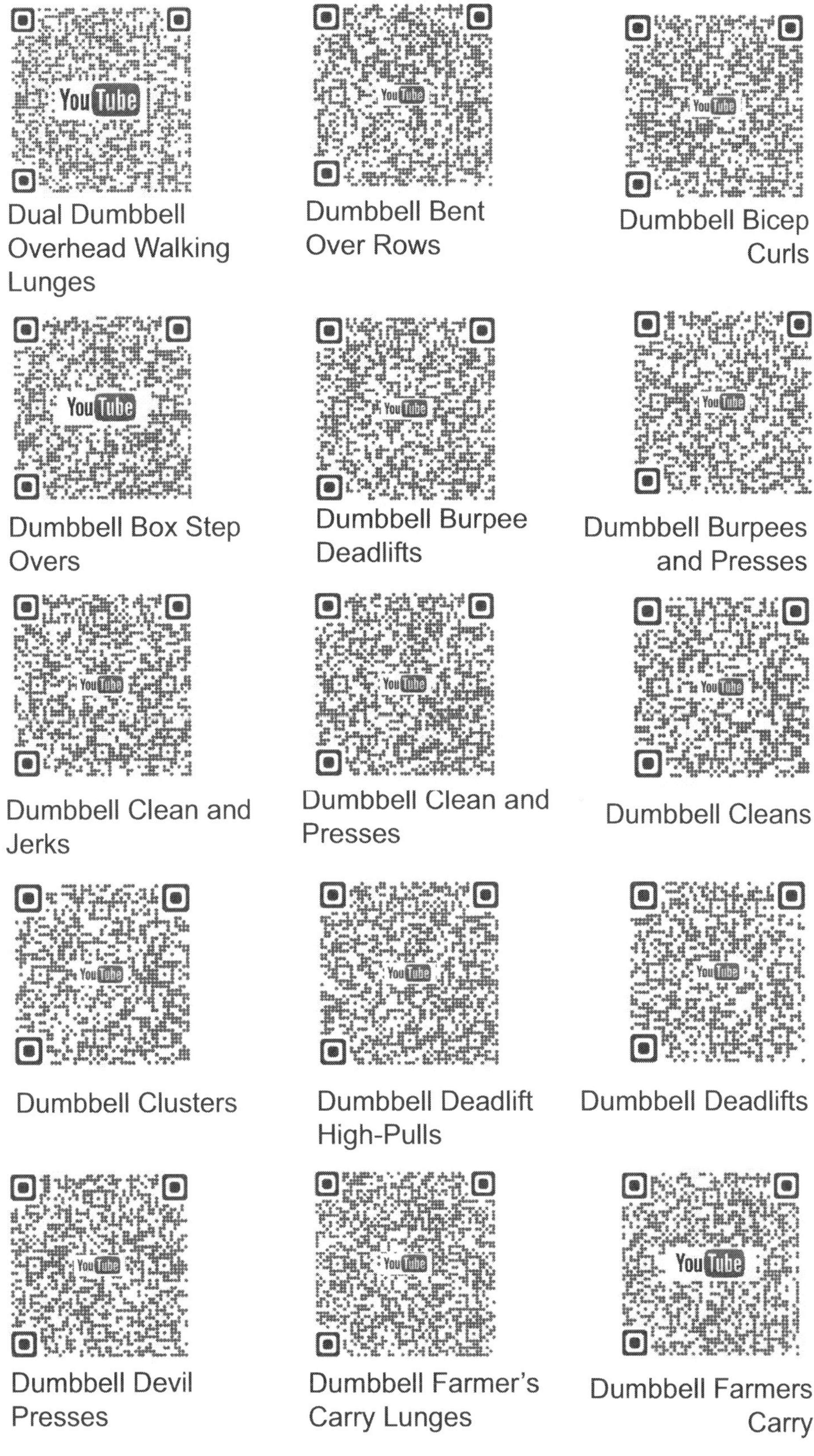

Dual Dumbbell Overhead Walking Lunges

Dumbbell Bent Over Rows

Dumbbell Bicep Curls

Dumbbell Box Step Overs

Dumbbell Burpee Deadlifts

Dumbbell Burpees and Presses

Dumbbell Clean and Jerks

Dumbbell Clean and Presses

Dumbbell Cleans

Dumbbell Clusters

Dumbbell Deadlift High-Pulls

Dumbbell Deadlifts

Dumbbell Devil Presses

Dumbbell Farmer's Carry Lunges

Dumbbell Farmers Carry

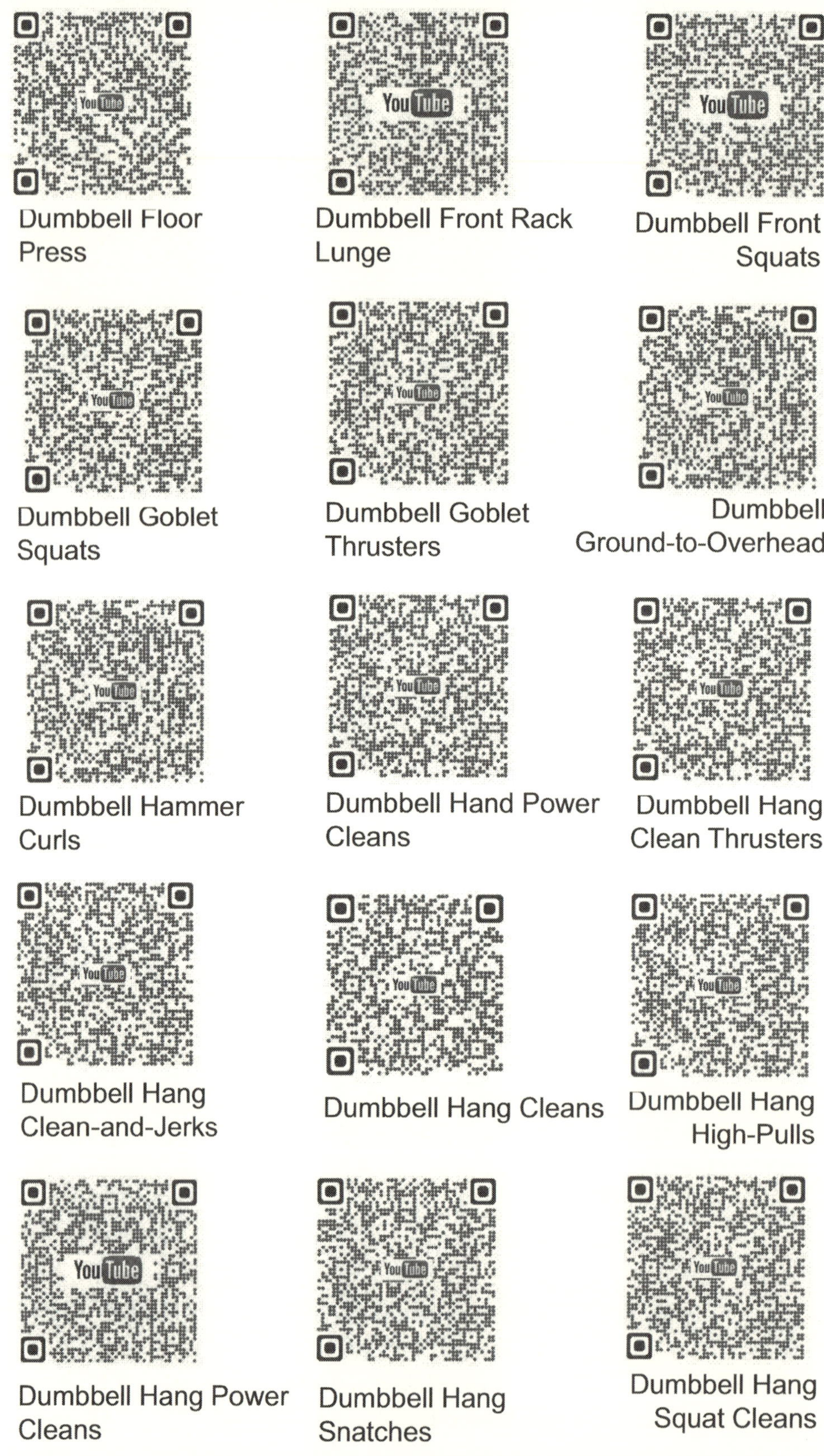

Dumbbell Floor Press

Dumbbell Front Rack Lunge

Dumbbell Front Squats

Dumbbell Goblet Squats

Dumbbell Goblet Thrusters

Dumbbell Ground-to-Overhead

Dumbbell Hammer Curls

Dumbbell Hand Power Cleans

Dumbbell Hang Clean Thrusters

Dumbbell Hang Clean-and-Jerks

Dumbbell Hang Cleans

Dumbbell Hang High-Pulls

Dumbbell Hang Power Cleans

Dumbbell Hang Snatches

Dumbbell Hang Squat Cleans

Dumbbell Hang Squat Thrusters

Dumbbell Lateral Raises

Dumbbell Lunges

Dumbbell Man-Makers

Dumbbell Overhead Lunges

Dumbbell Overhead Reverse Lunge

Dumbbell Overhead Lunge

Dumbbell Overhead Walking Lunges

Dumbbell Man Makers

Dumbbell Power Cleans

Dumbbell Push Jerks

Dumbbell Push Presses

Dumbbell Push-Ups

Dumbbell Push-up with Row

Dumbbell Reverse Lunges

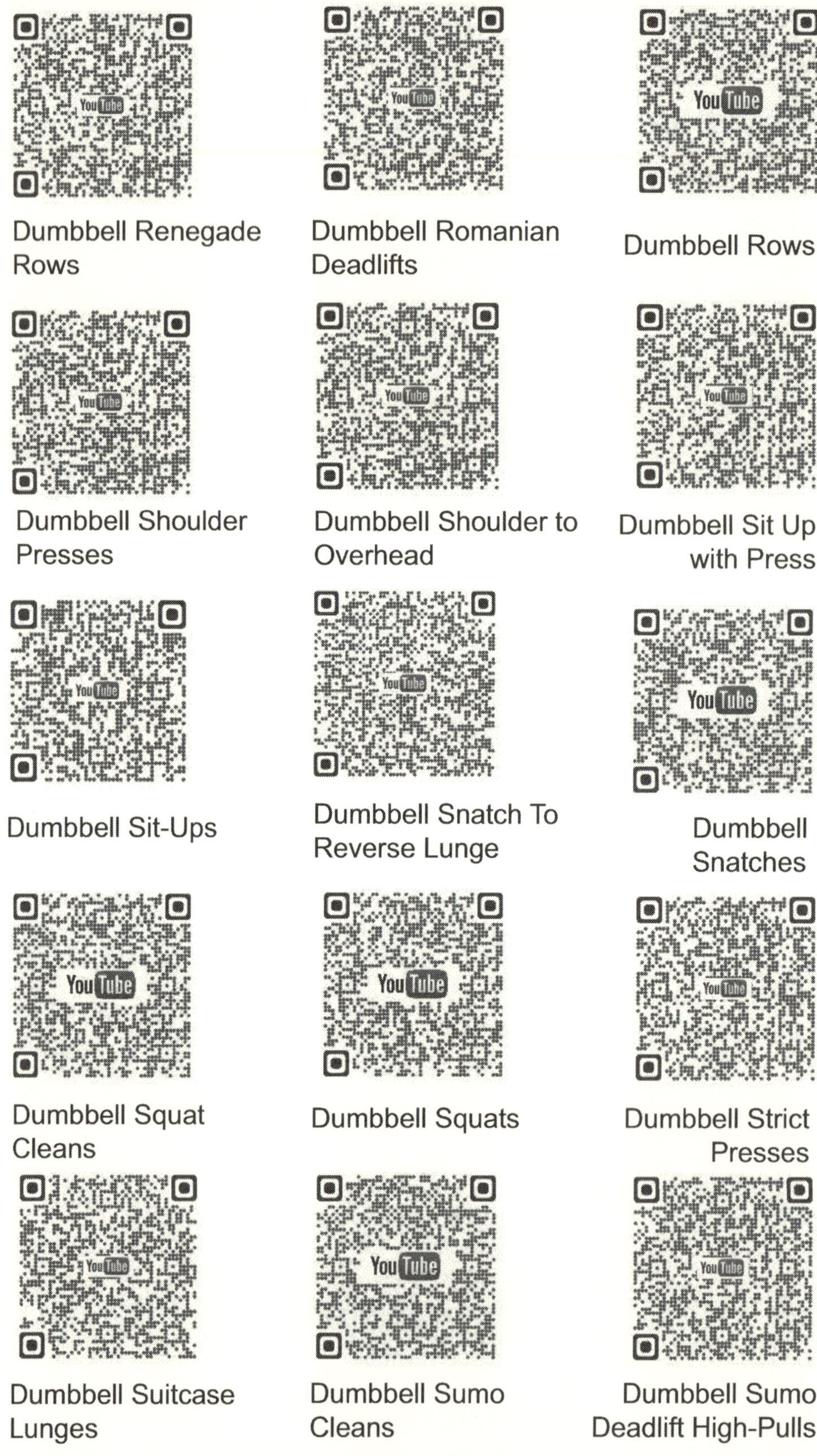

Dumbbell Renegade Rows

Dumbbell Romanian Deadlifts

Dumbbell Rows

Dumbbell Shoulder Presses

Dumbbell Shoulder to Overhead

Dumbbell Sit Up with Press

Dumbbell Sit-Ups

Dumbbell Snatch To Reverse Lunge

Dumbbell Snatches

Dumbbell Squat Cleans

Dumbbell Squats

Dumbbell Strict Presses

Dumbbell Suitcase Lunges

Dumbbell Sumo Cleans

Dumbbell Sumo Deadlift High-Pulls

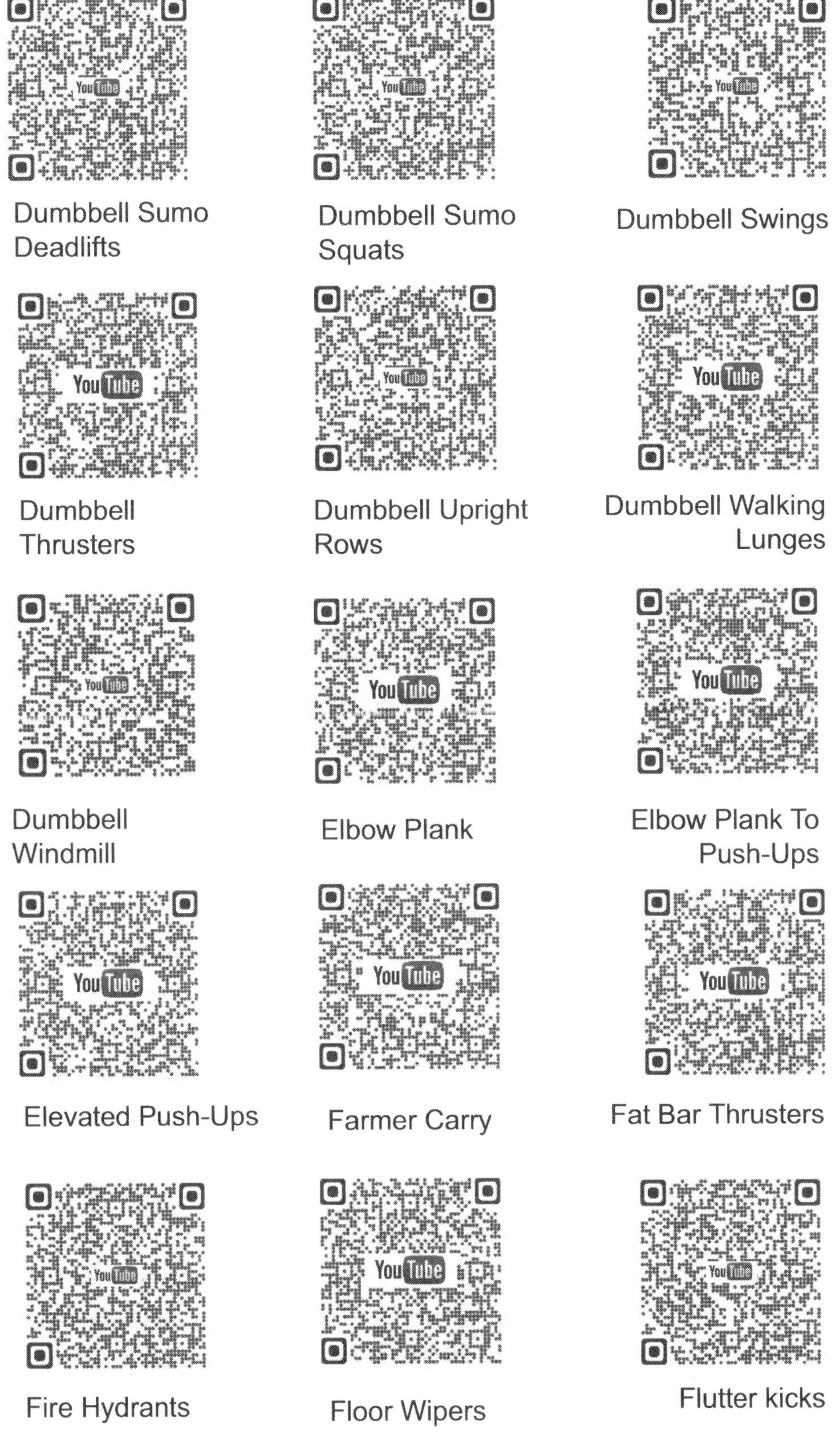

YouTube
Dumbbell Sumo Deadlifts
YouTube
Dumbbell Sumo Squats
YouTube
Dumbbell Swings
YouTube
Dumbbell Thrusters
YouTube
Dumbbell Upright Rows
YouTube
Dumbbell Walking Lunges
YouTube
Dumbbell Windmill
YouTube
Elbow Plank
YouTube
Elbow Plank To Push-Ups
YouTube
Elevated Push-Ups
YouTube
Farmer Carry
YouTube
Fat Bar Thrusters
YouTube
Fire Hydrants
YouTube
Floor Wipers
YouTube
Flutter kicks

Front Squats
Forward leg swings
Front kicks
Front lunges
GHD Sit-Ups
Glute bridges
Goblet Squats
Ground to Overheads
Half jacks
Hand Power Cleans
Hand Release Push-Ups
Hand to toe crunches
Handstand
Handstand Push-Ups
Handstand Walk

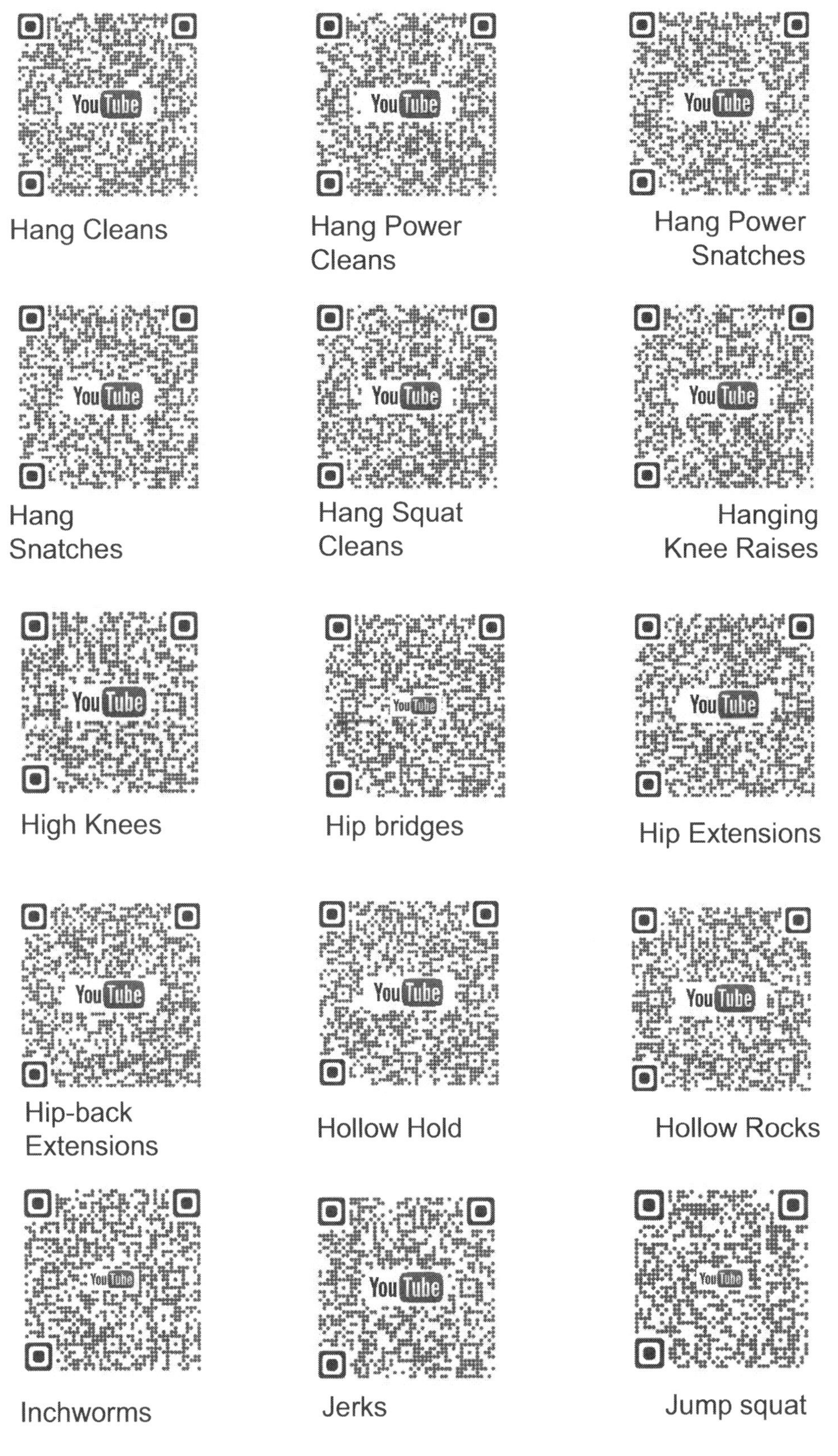

Hang Cleans

Hang Power Cleans

Hang Power Snatches

Hang Snatches

Hang Squat Cleans

Hanging Knee Raises

High Knees

Hip bridges

Hip Extensions

Hip-back Extensions

Hollow Hold

Hollow Rocks

Inchworms

Jerks

Jump squat

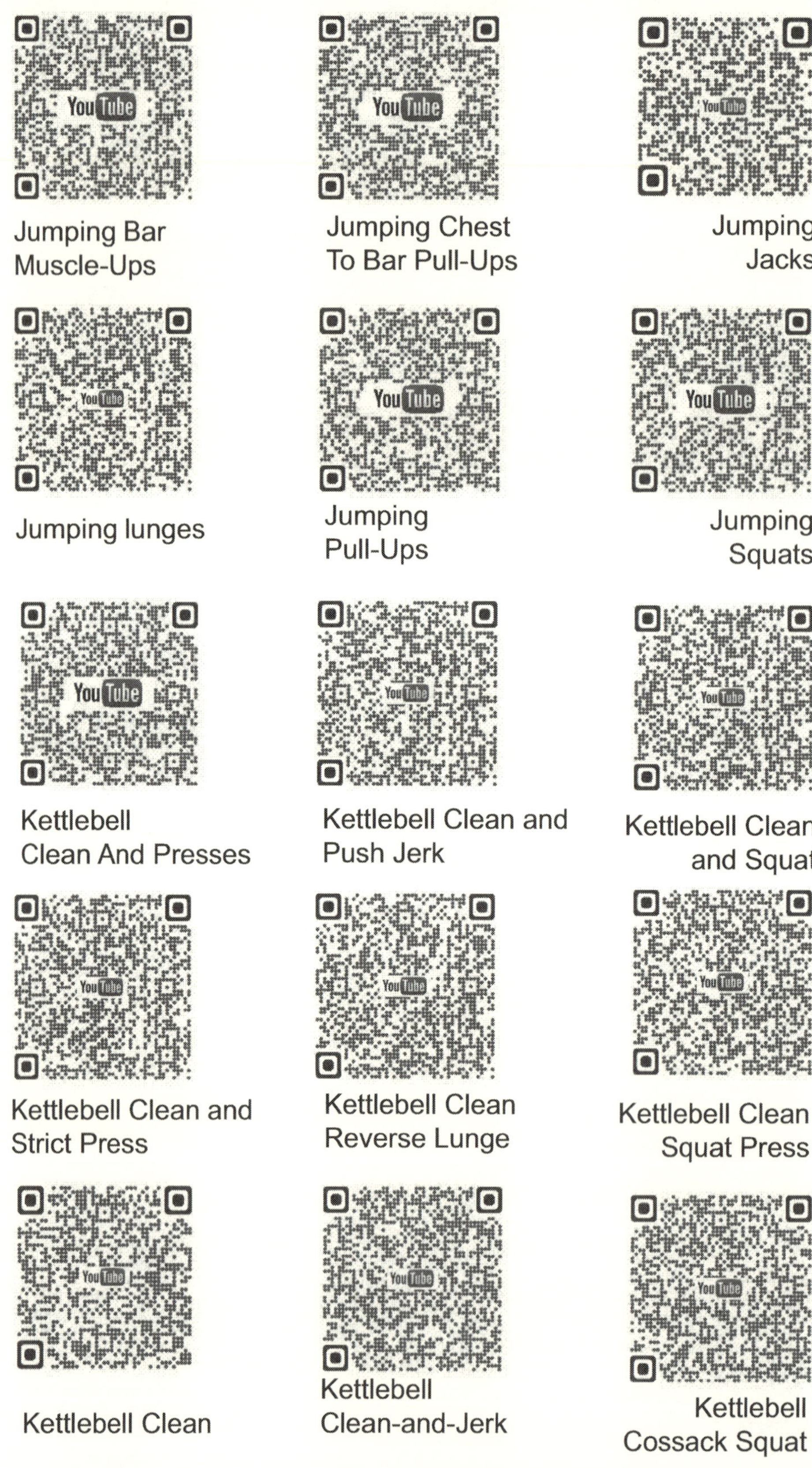

Jumping Bar Muscle-Ups

Jumping Chest To Bar Pull-Ups

Jumping Jacks

Jumping lunges

Jumping Pull-Ups

Jumping Squats

Kettlebell Clean And Presses

Kettlebell Clean and Push Jerk

Kettlebell Clean and Squat

Kettlebell Clean and Strict Press

Kettlebell Clean Reverse Lunge

Kettlebell Clean Squat Press

Kettlebell Clean

Kettlebell Clean-and-Jerk

Kettlebell Cossack Squat

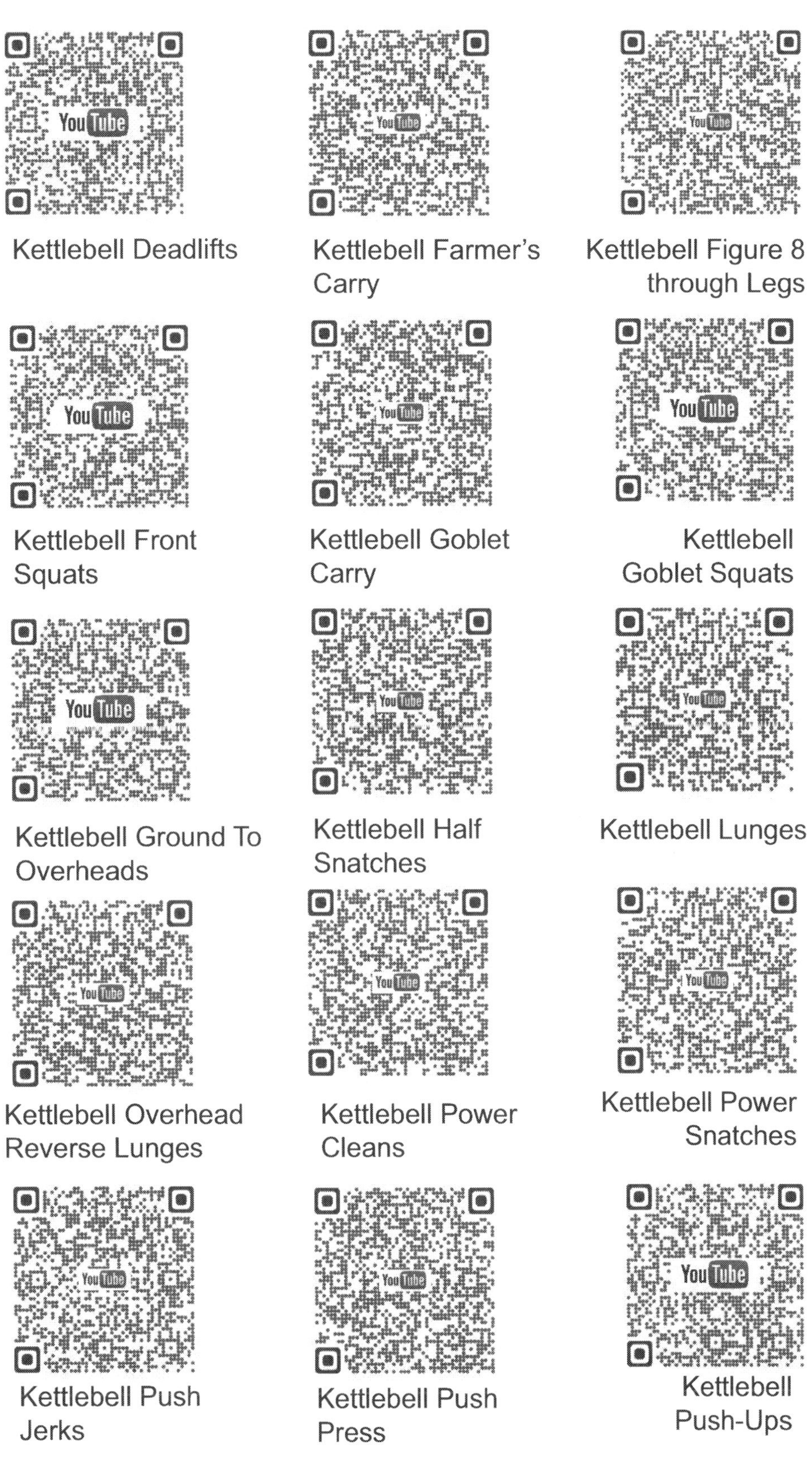

Kettlebell Deadlifts

Kettlebell Farmer's Carry

Kettlebell Figure 8 through Legs

Kettlebell Front Squats

Kettlebell Goblet Carry

Kettlebell Goblet Squats

Kettlebell Ground To Overheads

Kettlebell Half Snatches

Kettlebell Lunges

Kettlebell Overhead Reverse Lunges

Kettlebell Power Cleans

Kettlebell Power Snatches

Kettlebell Push Jerks

Kettlebell Push Press

Kettlebell Push-Ups

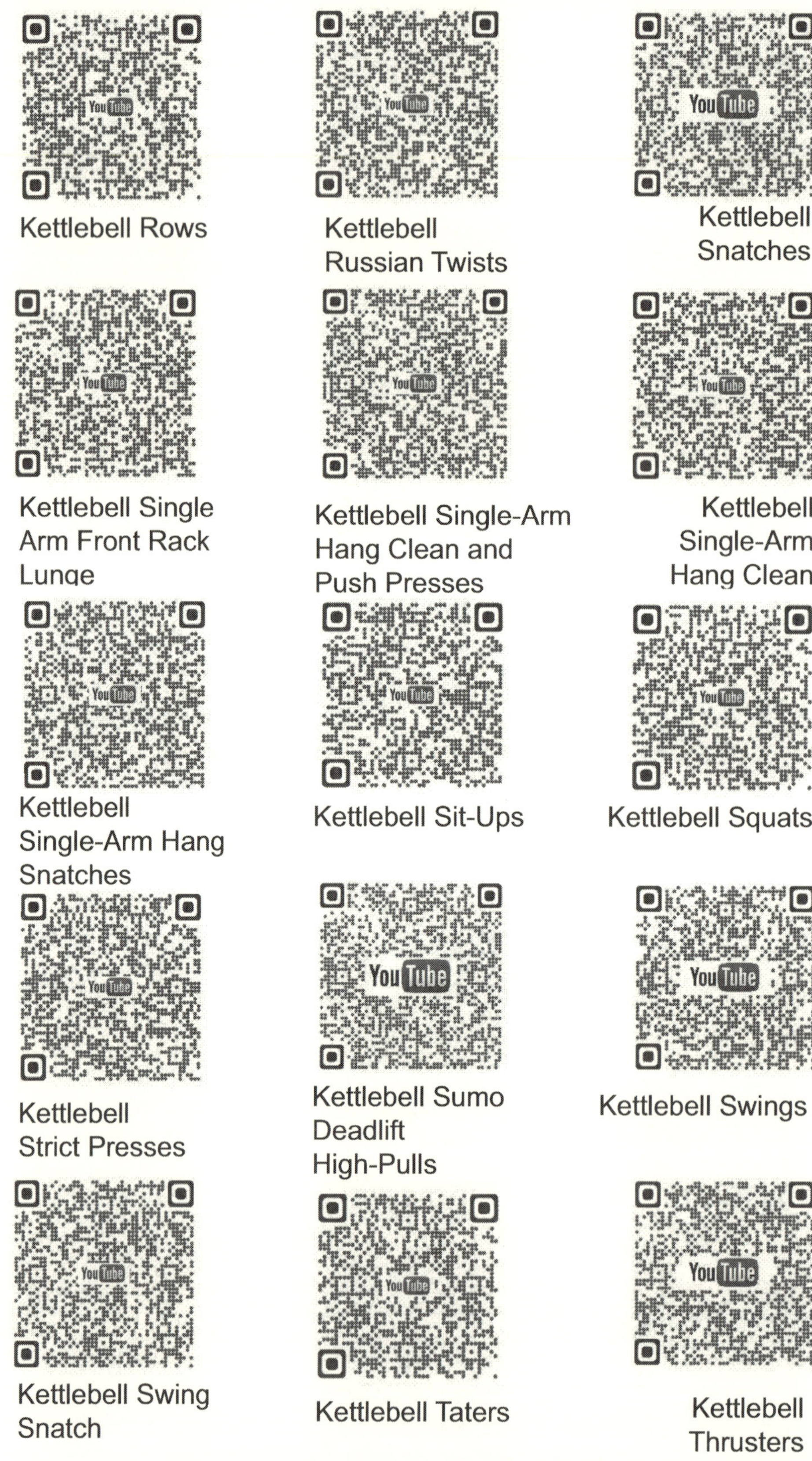

Kettlebell Rows

Kettlebell Russian Twists

Kettlebell Snatches

Kettlebell Single Arm Front Rack Lunge

Kettlebell Single-Arm Hang Clean and Push Presses

Kettlebell Single-Arm Hang Clean

Kettlebell Single-Arm Hang Snatches

Kettlebell Sit-Ups

Kettlebell Squats

Kettlebell Strict Presses

Kettlebell Sumo Deadlift High-Pulls

Kettlebell Swings

Kettlebell Swing Snatch

Kettlebell Taters

Kettlebell Thrusters

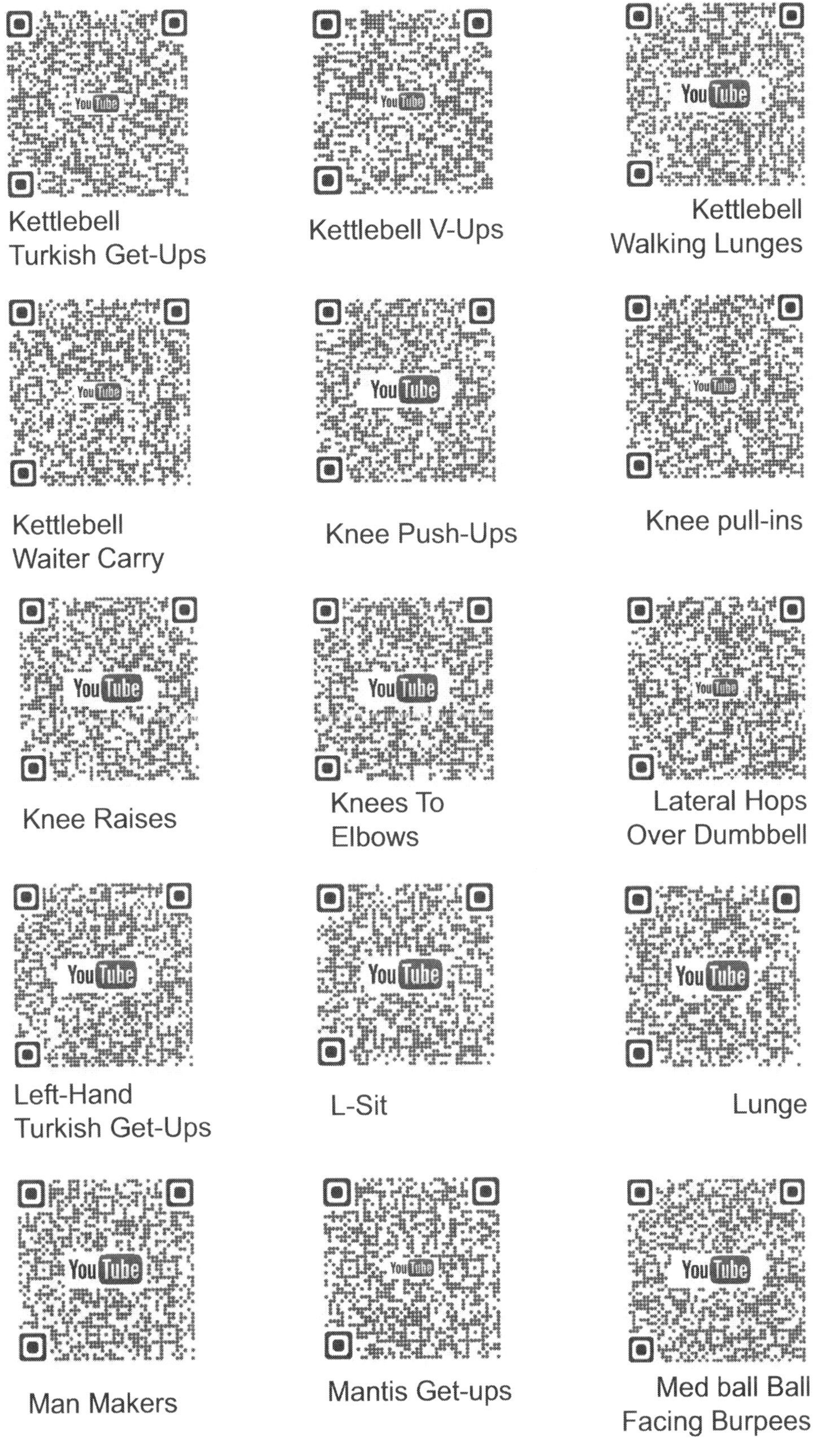

Kettlebell Turkish Get-Ups

Kettlebell V-Ups

Kettlebell Walking Lunges

Kettlebell Waiter Carry

Knee Push-Ups

Knee pull-ins

Knee Raises

Knees To Elbows

Lateral Hops Over Dumbbell

Left-Hand Turkish Get-Ups

L-Sit

Lunge

Man Makers

Mantis Get-ups

Med ball Ball Facing Burpees

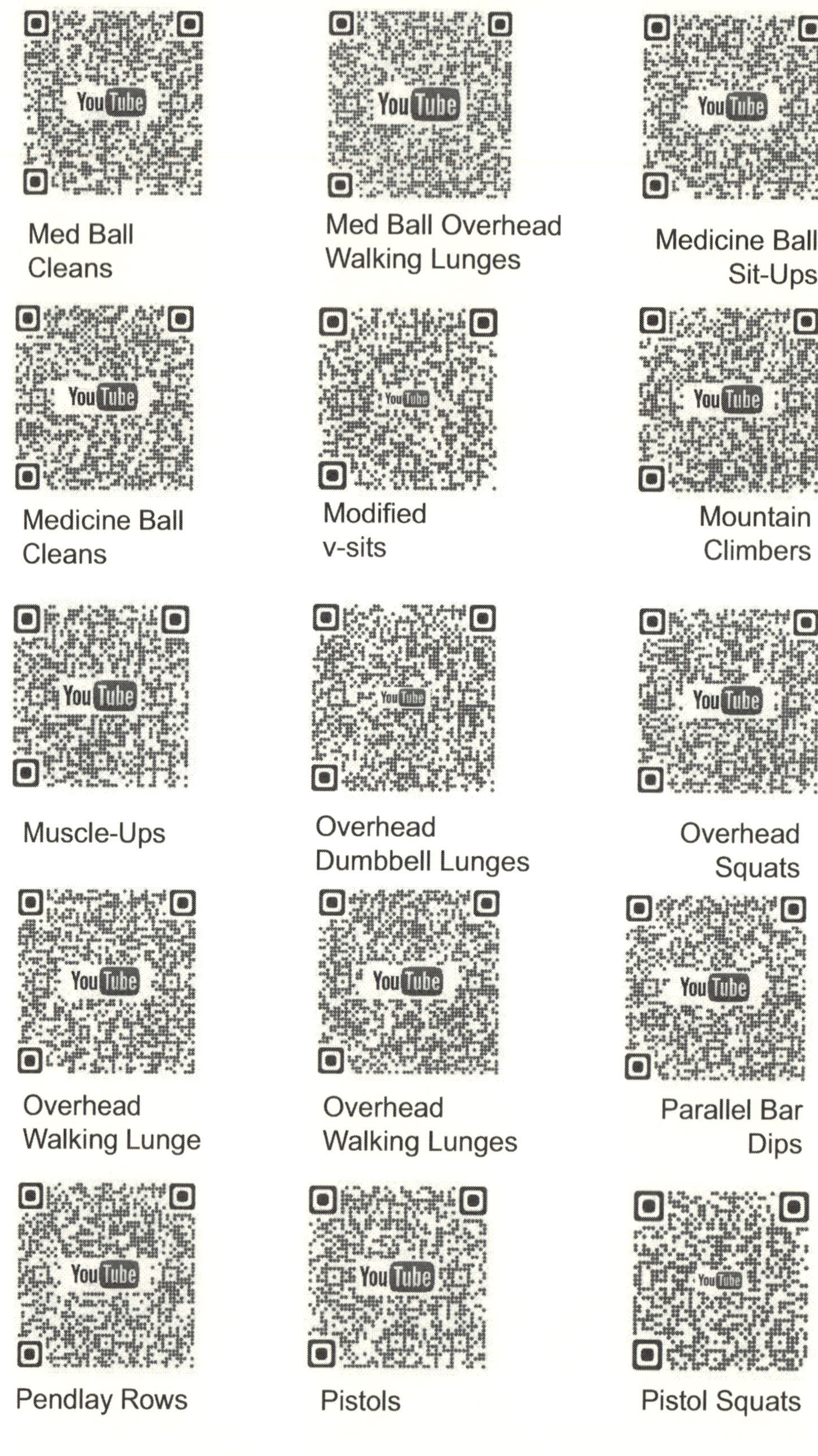

Med Ball Cleans

Med Ball Overhead Walking Lunges

Medicine Ball Sit-Ups

Medicine Ball Cleans

Modified v-sits

Mountain Climbers

Muscle-Ups

Overhead Dumbbell Lunges

Overhead Squats

Overhead Walking Lunge

Overhead Walking Lunges

Parallel Bar Dips

Pendlay Rows

Pistols

Pistol Squats

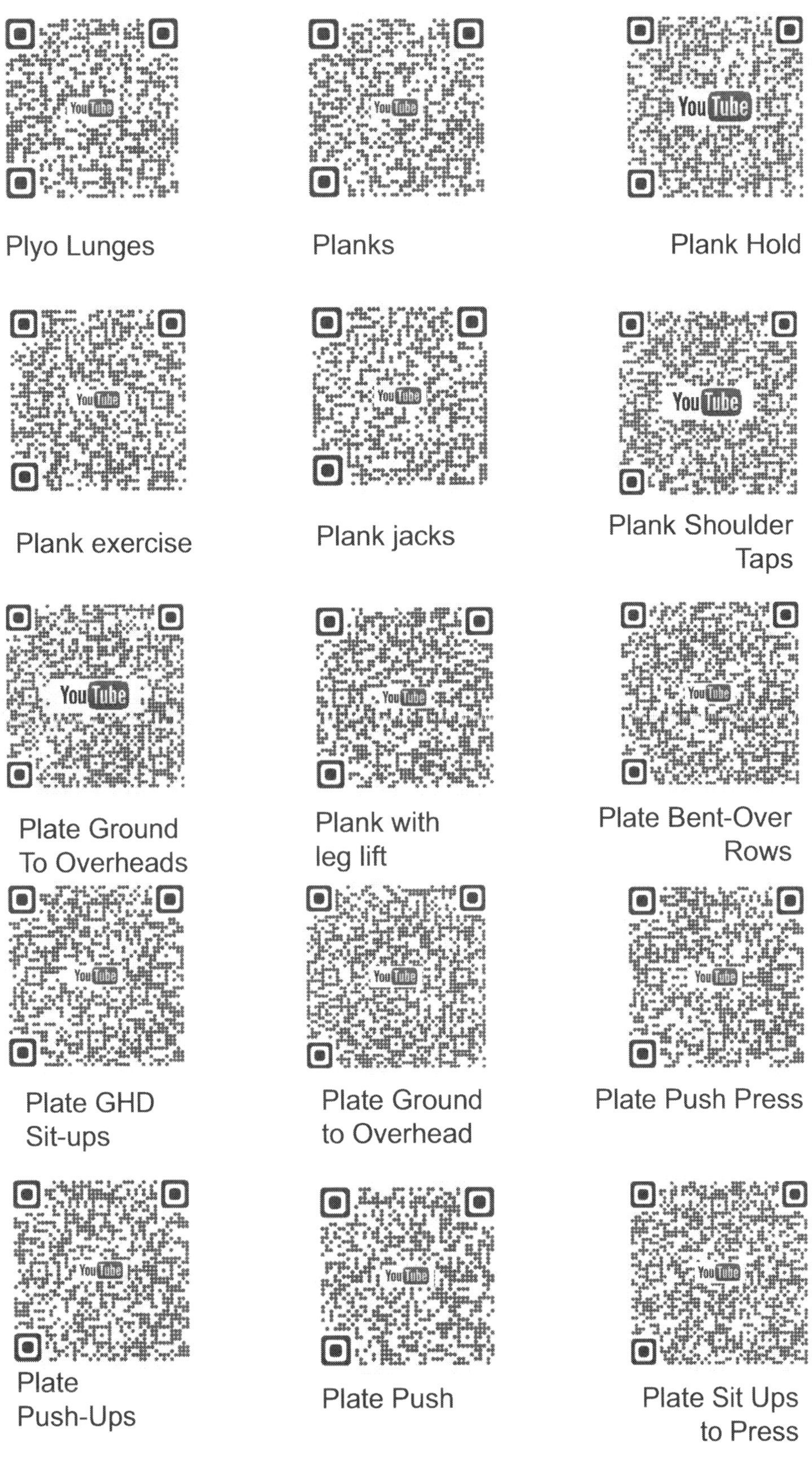

Plyo Lunges

Planks

Plank Hold

Plank exercise

Plank jacks

Plank Shoulder Taps

Plate Ground To Overheads

Plank with leg lift

Plate Bent-Over Rows

Plate GHD Sit-ups

Plate Ground to Overhead

Plate Push Press

Plate Push-Ups

Plate Push

Plate Sit Ups to Press

Plate Squats
Plate Overhead Lunges
Power Cleans
Power jacks
Power Snatches
Prison Squats
Pull-Ups
Push Jerks
Push Presses
Push-Ups
Push-ups with rotation
Raised leg circles
Renegade Rows
Reverse Bear Crawl
Reverse crunches

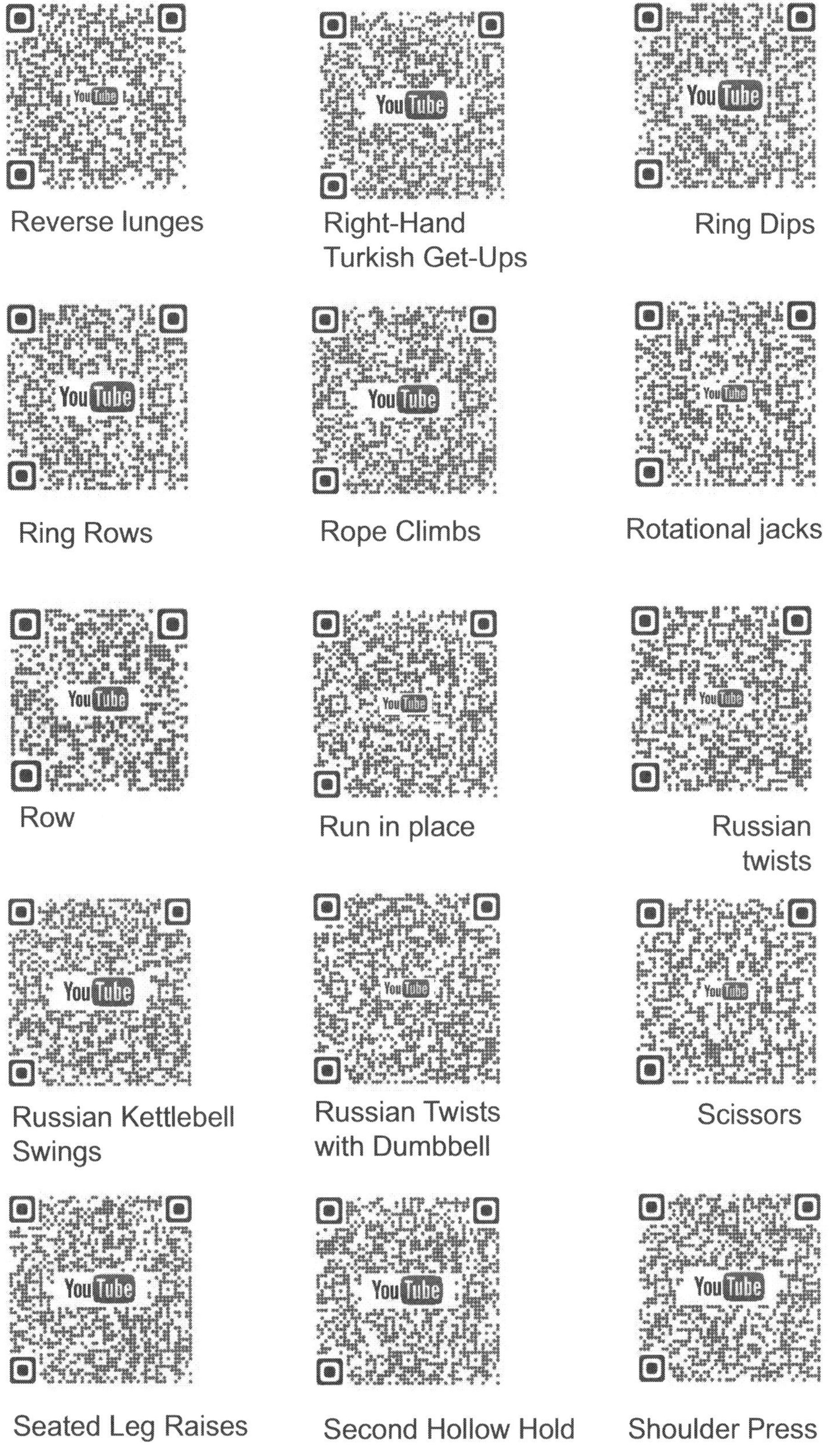

Reverse lunges

Right-Hand Turkish Get-Ups

Ring Dips

Ring Rows

Rope Climbs

Rotational jacks

Row

Run in place

Russian twists

Russian Kettlebell Swings

Russian Twists with Dumbbell

Scissors

Seated Leg Raises

Second Hollow Hold

Shoulder Press

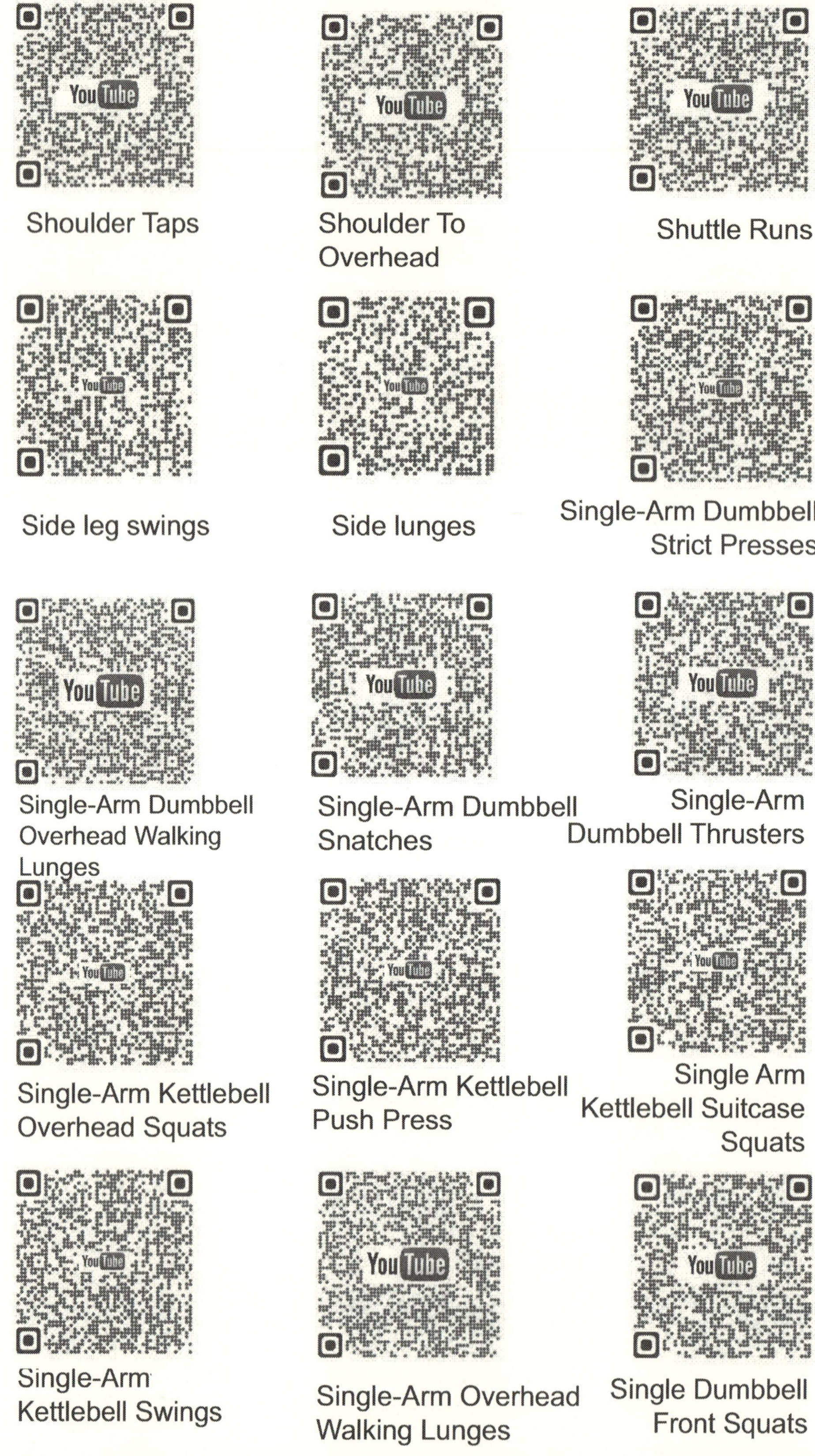
Shoulder Taps
Shoulder To Overhead
Shuttle Runs
Side leg swings
Side lunges
Single-Arm Dumbbell Strict Presses
Single-Arm Dumbbell Overhead Walking Lunges
Single-Arm Dumbbell Snatches
Single-Arm Dumbbell Thrusters
Single-Arm Kettlebell Overhead Squats
Single-Arm Kettlebell Push Press
Single Arm Kettlebell Suitcase Squats
Single-Arm Kettlebell Swings
Single-Arm Overhead Walking Lunges
Single Dumbbell Front Squats

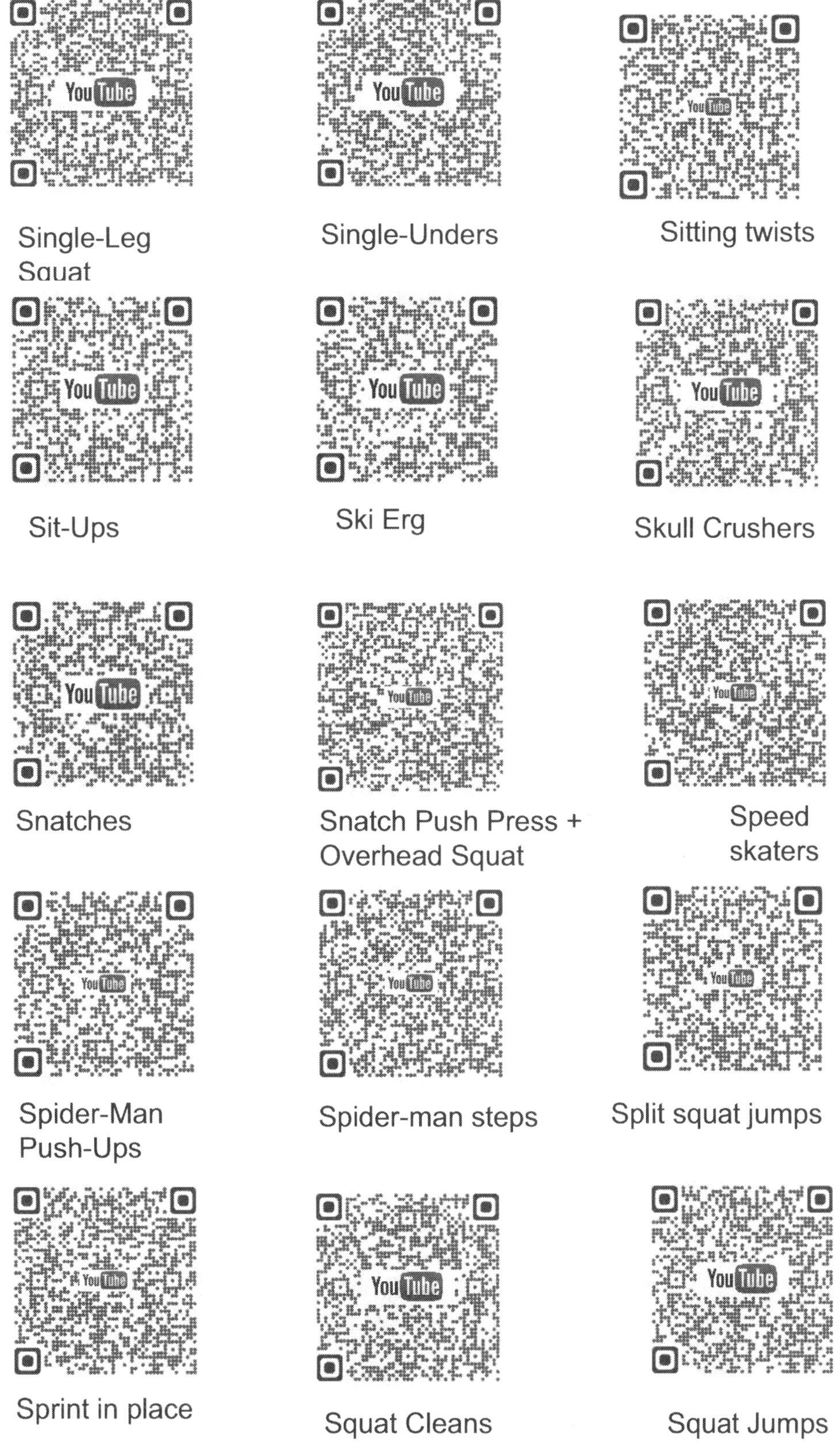
Single-Leg Squat
Single-Unders
Sitting twists
Sit-Ups
Ski Erg
Skull Crushers
Snatches
Snatch Push Press + Overhead Squat
Speed skaters
Spider-Man Push-Ups
Spider-man steps
Split squat jumps
Sprint in place
Squat Cleans
Squat Jumps

Squat to front kick
Squat Snatches
Squats
Step-Ups
Step ups exercise
Straight-leg donkey kick
Straight Leg Sit-Ups
Strict Chest-To Bar Pull-Ups
Strict Pull-Ups
Strict Ring Dips
Sumo Deadlift High Pulls
Sumo squats
Supermans
Supermans exercise
Thrusters

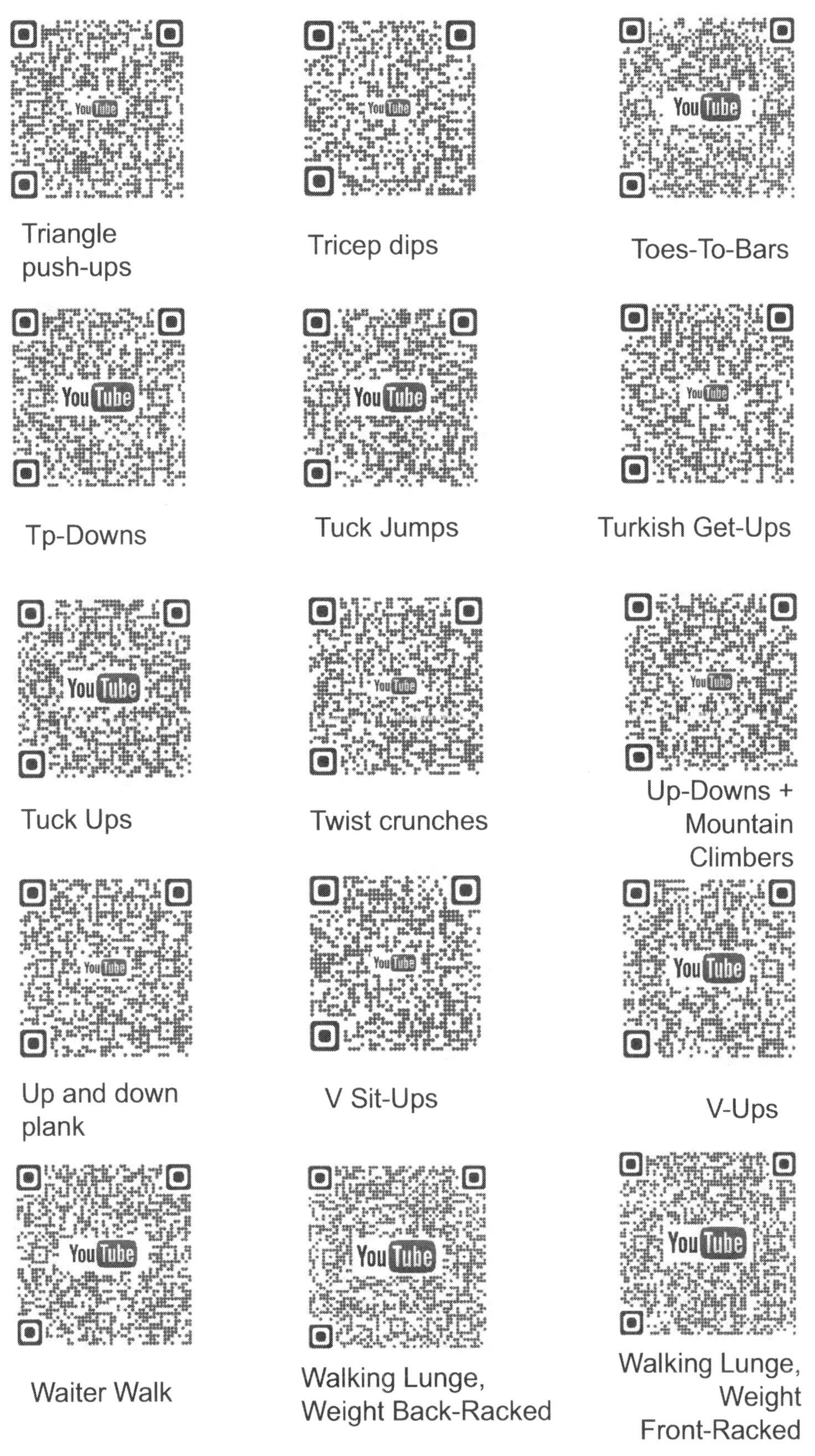
Triangle push-ups
Tricep dips
Toes-To-Bars
Tp-Downs
Tuck Jumps
Turkish Get-Ups
Tuck Ups
Twist crunches
Up-Downs + Mountain Climbers
Up and down plank
V Sit-Ups
V-Ups
Waiter Walk
Walking Lunge, Weight Back-Racked
Walking Lunge, Weight Front-Racked

Walking Lunge, Weight Overhead

Walking Lunge

Walking Lunge Steps

Walkouts To Push-Ups

Wall Ball Shots

Wall sit exercise

Wall Walk

Weighted Run

Windshield Wipers

Made in the USA
Las Vegas, NV
13 July 2023